EMERGENCY FIRST-AID
FUNDAMENTALS

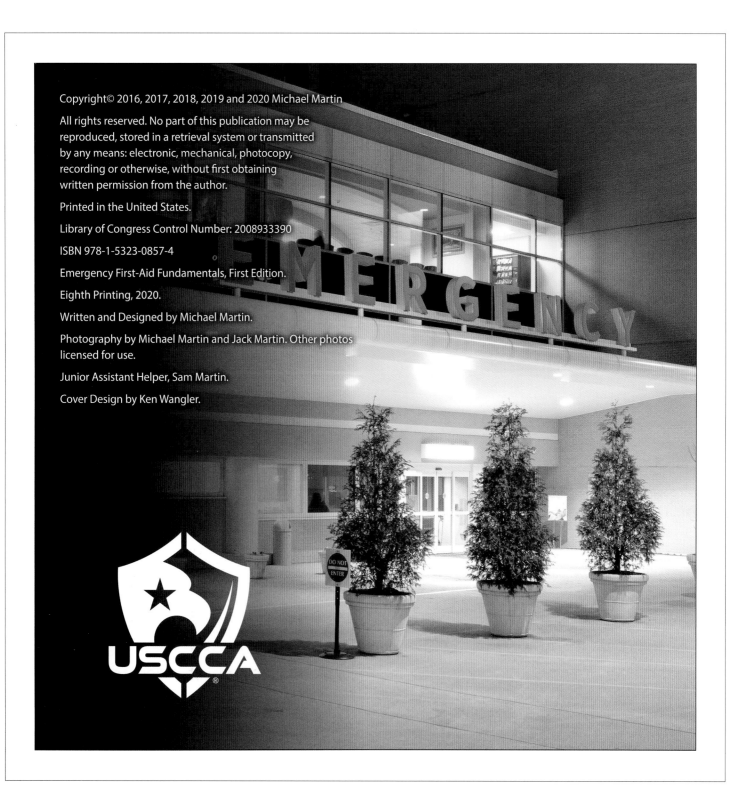

Printed in the United States.

Library of Congress Control Number: 2008933390

ISBN 978-1-5323-0857-4

Emergency First-Aid Fundamentals, First Edition.

Eighth Printing, 2020.

Written and Designed by Michael Martin.

Photography by Michael Martin and Jack Martin. Other photos licensed for use.

Junior Assistant Helper, Sam Martin.

Cover Design by Ken Wangler.

PREFACE

My team and I were about to begin the weekly checks of my station's fire engine and heavy rescue ladder when the call came in. As a member of my city's fire and EMS services, I'd grown to realize that most of our calls lacked the excitement portrayed in TV dramas centered around the fire service. But every once in a while, a call comes in that raises the hair on the back of our necks, and this was one of those calls. Even beyond structure fires and car crashes, one particular call always guarantees that life is hanging in the balance. The calls for a victim in cardiac arrest. The call on that particular day came in on what had otherwise been a relatively quiet day. Even before the dispatcher finished with the details of the call, my partner had jumped into the driver's seat of our ambulance as I swung into the front right seat. I checked us into service, hit the lights and siren, and quickly used our mapping software to give us the quickest route. I was relieved to see that we were within three minutes of the incident, and our lights and siren would ensure a clear path through the midmorning traffic. After arriving on the scene moments later, my partner and I jumped out of the rig to grab our gear, and we were joined by two police officers who had arrived just seconds after us. Bolting through the door, we were directed to the victim by a bystander, and according to our official report of the call, we had our LUCAS device attached within 90 seconds, with a secure airway placed moments after that. As one crew member provided ventilations to the patient and the LUCAS provided mechanical chest compressions, my partner and I connected the patient to our cardiac monitor, shocks were delivered, an IV was placed, and we started the flow of critical medications designed to restart the patient's heart. A bystander watching us might have been convinced that he or she was watching a choreographed scene, and in a way, it *was* choreographed. Each of us knew our specific roles and we knew them incredibly well. Everything on that scene went exactly as it was supposed go. And yet, the patient died.

Less than two weeks later, another crew from my station got a call that was eerily similar. The patient was about the same age, and the ambulance crew arrived on scene at about the same three-minute mark. Their scene would have been a carbon copy of ours, with the LUCAS being attached within 90 seconds of arriving at the side of the victim, and a secure airway being placed seconds after that. An IV and meds would have been started, the electrical signals in the patient's heart would have been analyzed, and shocks would have been delivered. Everything would have been choreographed the same as our scene. Yet, that patient survived.

While you might be tempted to write the different outcomes off to fate, the truth is, there was one *dramatic* difference between our two scenes. But the difference had nothing to do with how our two EMS crews responded upon arrival at the respective scenes. The difference was what the bystanders did *before* we arrived. On my scene, the bystanders were unable or unwilling to begin CPR, so my patient's heart remained idle for the five minutes between the time the 911 call was made and the time when we started compressions. On the second scene, as one bystander called 911, other bystanders began to immediately provide hard and deep chest compressions. Those five minutes of bystander action (or inaction) very likely made the difference between the two outcomes. While those two cases touched me personally, there are literally tens of thousands of cases every year where bystanders make the difference between life and death simply by bridging the gap between the start of the incident and the arrival of EMS to the scene. As I'll mention to the Cub Scout and Boy Scout groups that visit my fire station, after calling 911, the most common next step that bystanders take is to do nothing. While the goal of this book isn't to turn you into a field surgeon or to bring your skill level to that of a trained and licensed paramedic or EMT, it *is* designed to give you the practical knowledge to know what the next steps should be after calling 911 and to bridge the gap between your arrival on the scene and the arrival of EMS.

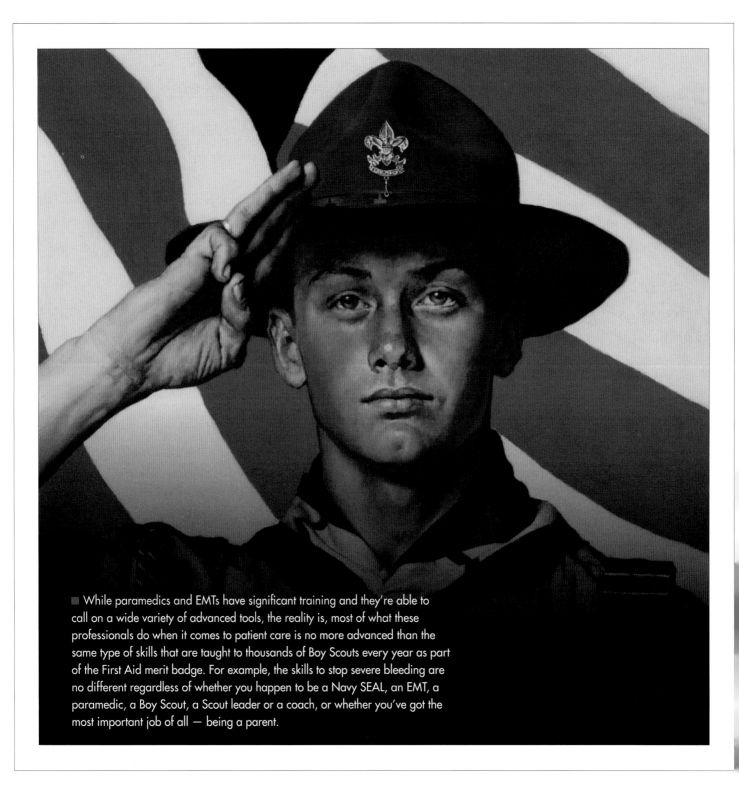

While paramedics and EMTs have significant training and they're able to call on a wide variety of advanced tools, the reality is, most of what these professionals do when it comes to patient care is no more advanced than the same type of skills that are taught to thousands of Boy Scouts every year as part of the First Aid merit badge. For example, the skills to stop severe bleeding are no different regardless of whether you happen to be a Navy SEAL, an EMT, a paramedic, a Boy Scout, a Scout leader or a coach, or whether you've got the most important job of all — being a parent.

INTRODUCTION

Would you know what to do if you were deep in the wilderness and a hunting companion sustained a penetrating chest wound from an errant round? Could you prolong the life of a loved one long enough for the ambulance to arrive, if he or she had sustained a lacerated artery from a violent attacker armed with a knife? Could you take charge of a scene and bridge the gap between the start of the emergency and the arrival of EMS for a patient suffering from cardiac arrest, a fractured femur, an anaphylactic reaction or a diabetic emergency? While most Americans are comfortable dealing with the cuts and scrapes of everyday life and tens of thousands have learned the Heimlich maneuver and CPR, most individuals would be a bit *less* comfortable dealing with severe, life-threatening injuries or illnesses when seconds count and EMS and the emergency room are minutes (or longer) away. The goal of this book is to help you gain the knowledge, confidence and competence needed to deal with dozens of medical and traumatic emergencies, including each of those mentioned.

That knowledge will include knowing what to do if you are ever confronted with a loved one falling victim to cardiac arrest or another significant life threat, such as severe arterial bleeding, a gunshot wound, a significant burn injury, a diabetic emergency, stroke, shock or a number of other traumatic and medical emergencies. While severe bleeding or a significant burn might be an

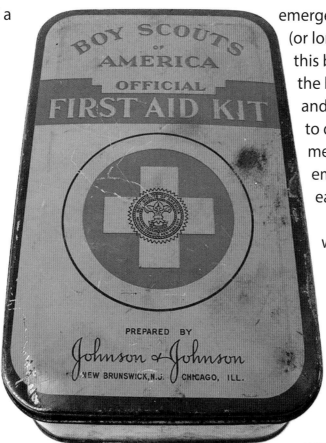

■ Some Things Never Change
While treatments, diagnostic tools and medical devices have radically changed over the years, in some ways, the fundamentals of emergency care haven't changed much since the Boy Scouts of America partnered with Johnson & Johnson to create this "Boy Scouts of America Official First Aid Kit" in the 1930s. The sterile gauze packed in this kit would be as effective at stopping severe bleeding today as it was more than 80 years ago.

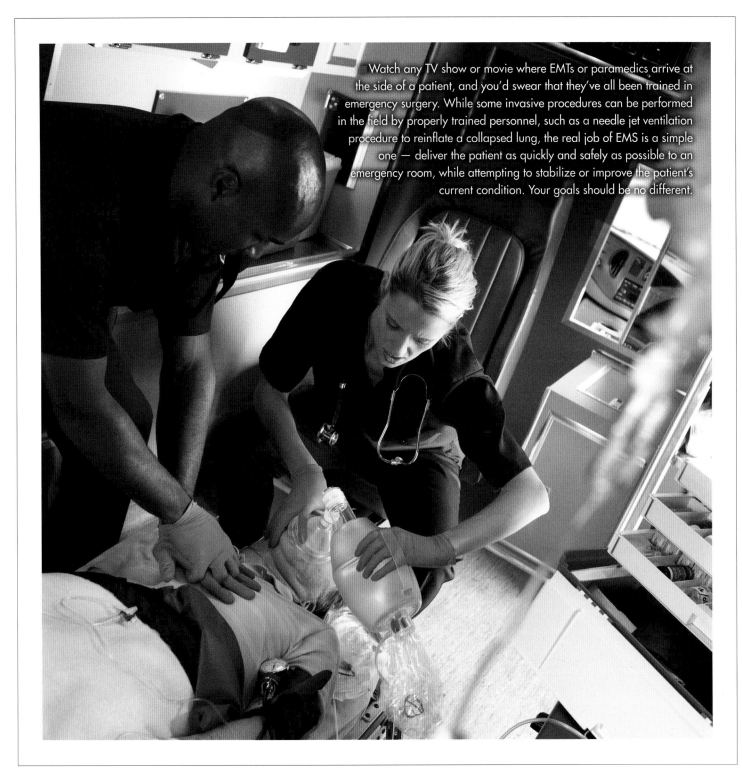

Watch any TV show or movie where EMTs or paramedics arrive at the side of a patient, and you'd swear that they've all been trained in emergency surgery. While some invasive procedures can be performed in the field by properly trained personnel, such as a needle jet ventilation procedure to reinflate a collapsed lung, the real job of EMS is a simple one — deliver the patient as quickly and safely as possible to an emergency room, while attempting to stabilize or improve the patient's current condition. Your goals should be no different.

easy thing to diagnose, this book will also focus on helping you understand a number of signs and symptoms for a variety of conditions, and to guide you on which course of action you should take. In many cases, properly assessing a patient will lead you to make specific interventions using a specific set of tools or skills that will be covered in this book, but in other cases, understanding the signs and symptoms of a particular medical condition, such as a stroke, will lead you to the only intervention that will make a difference, namely, getting your patient to EMS or getting EMS to your patient as quickly as possible.

While you might assume that the interventions, tools and skills that I'll be reviewing in this book will be radically different than those used by professional EMTs and paramedics, that's actually not the case. While some advanced procedures can be performed in the field by properly trained personnel, such as a needle jet ventilation procedure used to reinflate a collapsed lung, the real job of EMS is a simple one — to deliver the patient as quickly and as safely as possible to an emergency room, while attempting to stabilize or improve the patient's current condition. Your goals should be no different.

While there is a lot that professionals and non-professionals have in common,

one interesting difference is that, in certain situations, nonprofessionals might have to perform additional tasks that even the pros don't need to accomplish. That difference lies in whether a patient's condition must simply be corrected or whether it must be corrected, and then maintained. Let me explain that last sentence a bit further: When EMS personnel arrive on a scene, they have the luxury of knowing that, even for the most serious medical or traumatic emergencies, the emergency room might be no more than 30 minutes away, and it's often much closer than that. That means that they can remain focused on correcting any major life threats and correcting deficiencies to their patient's ABCs, while being less concerned with the maintenance of the condition. For example, in a case of severe bleeding, EMS personnel will be concerned with stopping the bleeding and monitoring and/or treating their patient for shock. They won't concern themselves with intense cleansing of the wound to ward off infection, and they won't attempt to close the wound using something like adhesive sutures. On the other hand, nonprofessionals might find themselves hours or even days from the emergency room. Outside of urban and suburban areas, millions of U.S. citizens are outside of the "golden hour" of EMS arrival, and if you've embarked on a camping, hiking or canoe trip, you might find yourself literally days from EMS support and the entrance to the emergency room. That might mean that, as a nonprofessional, you'll need to conduct a few tasks that even the guys in the back of the ambulance don't do on a regular basis. Don't worry. I'll not only cover in detail what you'll need to think about for the first hour of a medical or traumatic emergency; I'll also cover what you'll need to consider if that hour stretches into days. It all starts with a good assessment, and that's where Chapter 1 comes in.

Chapter 1 begins with an explanation of how to conduct a patient and scene assessment, including a primary assessment, an assessment of the patient's ABCs and a secondary (or rapid trauma) assessment. I'll modify the steps of the assessment slightly from what I'll use when I'm on duty, but the fact is, most of the assessment checklist applies regardless of your level of training. For example, the first item on the primary assessment checklist is to determine scene safety — that's an important checkpoint regardless of your level of training. The primary and secondary assessments continue through a methodical checklist, including (but not limited to) evaluating your patient for immediate life threats (all of which will be covered in Chapters 2 and 3), evaluating your patient's ABCs, determining the need for spinal immobilization and knowing how to perform a rapid trauma assessment to find traumatic injuries not previously detected.

Chapters 2 and 3 will go on to introduce you to a wide variety of life-threatening traumatic and medical conditions. Those chapters are laid out in an easy-to-understand format. Each section will begin with an overview of that particular traumatic or medical condition, including an explanation of the signs and symptoms that might be discovered during your assessment. Some conditions will be easy to diagnose, such as severe arterial bleeding, while some will be more nuanced, such as a diabetic emergency or a stroke, and might be mistaken for another condition. Following signs and symptoms, I'll discuss the field treatment for each condition, including easy-to-follow, step-by-step instructions and photos where appropriate. Chapter 2 focuses entirely on traumatic emergencies, including severe arterial bleeding, maintenance of a severe laceration, penetrating chest injuries, severe burns, musculoskeletal trauma, femur fractures, pelvis fractures, simple and complex rib fractures, head trauma, and trauma to the eye. Chapter 3's focus is on medical emergencies, including myocardial infarctions (heart attacks), cardiac arrest, diabetic

MODERN EMERGENCY MEDICAL SERVICES
HOW PREHOSPITAL CARE EVOLVED FROM THE LOCAL UNDERTAKER TO MODERN, ON-SCENE EMERGENCY CARE

Until the late 1960s and early '70s, prehospital care was largely unregulated and was managed by services as diverse as hospital interns driving horse-drawn carriages to the local undertaker delivering patients to the hospital in a hearse. That all changed in 1966, when the National Academy of Sciences National Research Council published a white paper titled *Accidental Death and Disability: The Neglected Disease of Modern Society*. The paper laid bare the deficiencies of prehospital care and made a number of recommendations for the standardization of

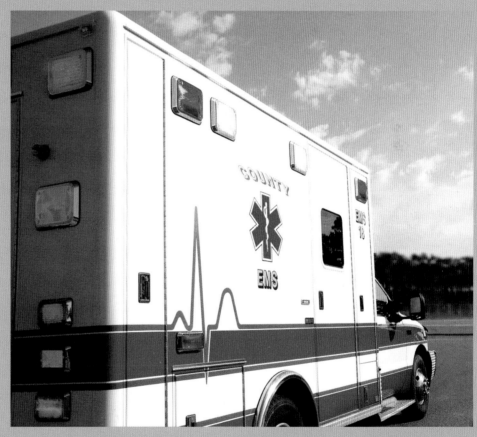

ambulance services and the training of prehospital providers. In today's society, prehospital care is managed by a sophisticated network of basic and advanced life services (BLS and ALS), requiring certification by national and state registries. On a typical ambulance call today, patients should expect to see at least one ALS provider (a paramedic) and one BLS provider (an EMT or Emergency Medical Technician) capable of providing sophisticated prehospital care from the moment they arrive on scene until the moment that the patient is handed off to emergency room staff.

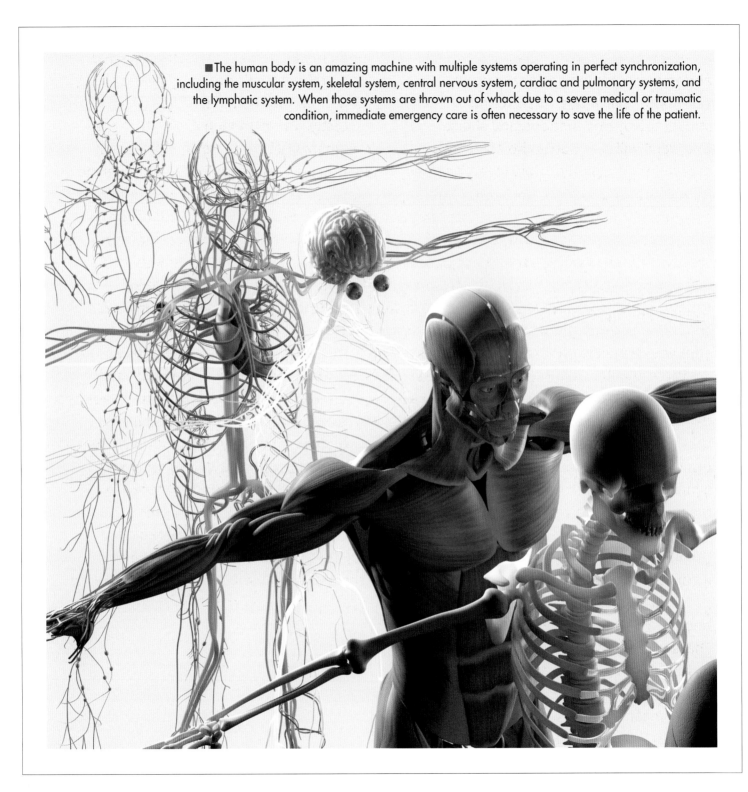

The human body is an amazing machine with multiple systems operating in perfect synchronization, including the muscular system, skeletal system, central nervous system, cardiac and pulmonary systems, and the lymphatic system. When those systems are thrown out of whack due to a severe medical or traumatic condition, immediate emergency care is often necessary to save the life of the patient.

emergencies, stroke, seizures and syncope, abdominal emergencies, anaphylaxis, venomous snakebites, hypothermia, heat stroke, airway obstructions, and shock. Chapter 4 will summarize the book with everything you should know when it comes to building your own emergency first-aid kit for a variety of conditions. In that chapter, I'll also review a number of my favorite off-the-shelf trauma kits, plus some other gear and gadgets that have found their way into my own emergency first-aid kits. I'll end that chapter with some suggestions on what to do after you've finished this book.

Three final notes before we get started: You'll notice that, throughout the book, I've defined a number of medical terms (these will show up in a blue box), including the proper pronunciation. I've done that any time I use a medical term that isn't used in common practice, including words like hypoperfusion, cyanosis, distal, pneumothorax and others. You'll know what all of those terms (and more) mean by the end of the book.

You'll also notice that, throughout the book, I refer to the victim as "your patient." That's not to imply that you suddenly have an MD or RN following your name (assuming you don't have one there already) but what it *does* mean is that, from the moment you assume a leadership role at the scene to the moment EMS arrives (or another bystander with a higher level of training relieves you), the victim *is* your patient.

Lastly, it's worth mentioning that the treatments I'll be discussing in this book are not a substitute for EMS or emergency room care. In other words, the treatments I'll discuss are meant to extend the life of your patient so that you'll be able to reach EMS support and the emergency room, not so that you can skip them altogether. While many of the treatments will be critical even if EMS is minutes away, such as starting CPR or stopping severe arterial bleeding, other treatments, such as closing a wound with adhesive sutures, will only be necessary if EMS and the emergency room are hours or days away.

While this book won't teach you how to perform an emergency tracheotomy with a pocketknife and a ball-point pen, it will teach you to save the life of a critically injured or ill patient when seconds count and EMS and the emergency room are minutes (or longer) away.

CONTENTS

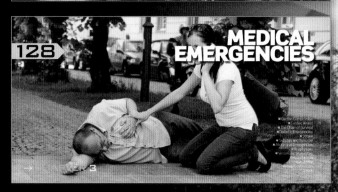
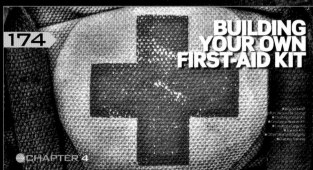

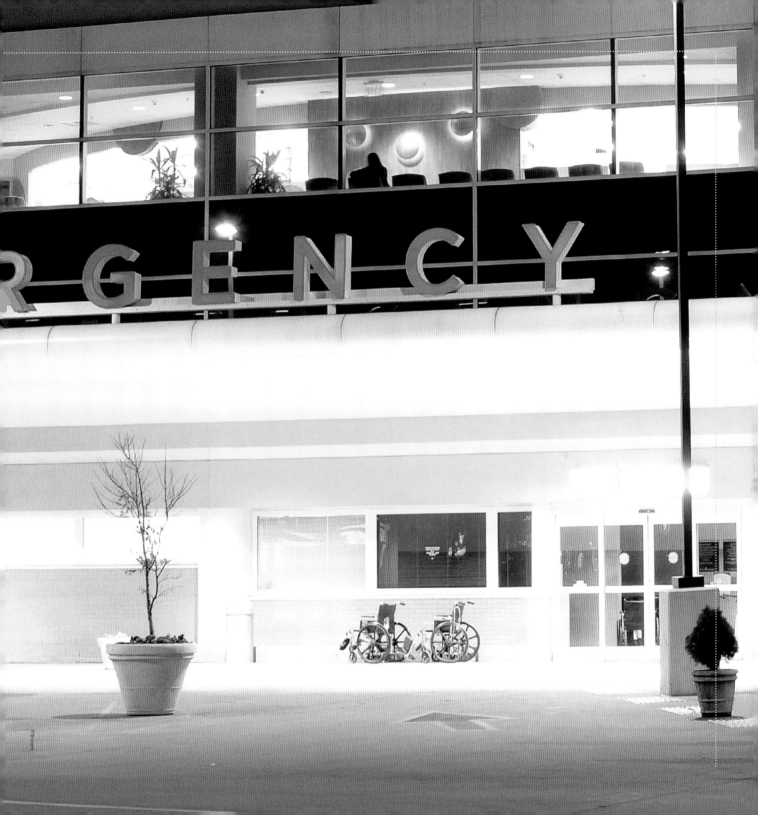

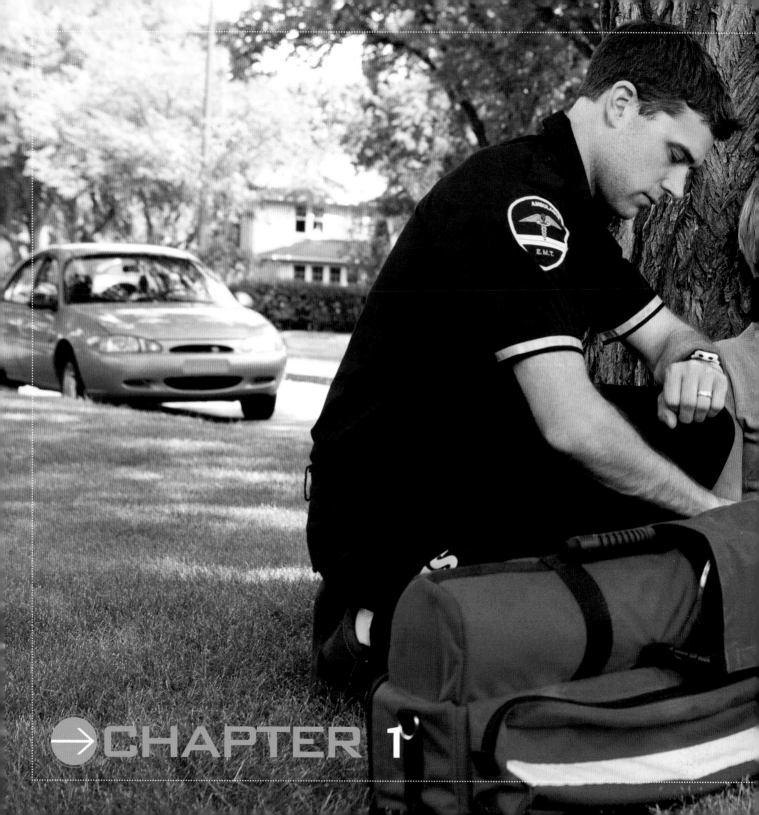

CHAPTER 1

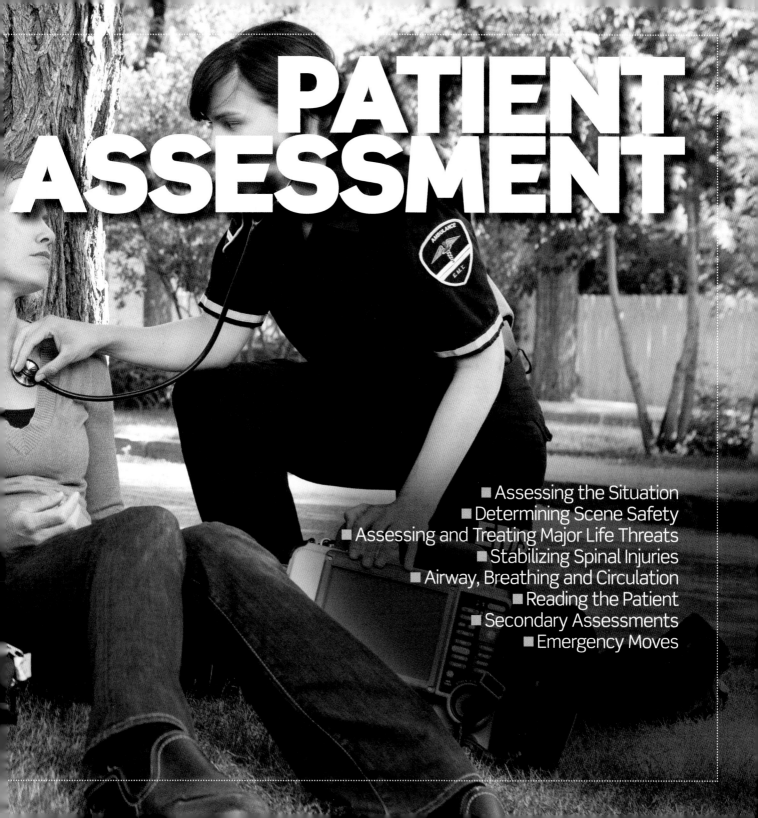

PATIENT ASSESSMENT

- Assessing the Situation
- Determining Scene Safety
- Assessing and Treating Major Life Threats
- Stabilizing Spinal Injuries
- Airway, Breathing and Circulation
- Reading the Patient
- Secondary Assessments
- Emergency Moves

A common thread exists in all first-responder education, regardless of whether that education is for police officers, firefighters, paramedics or EMTs. How to assess a situation is at the top of the list of things to learn. Assessing the safety of the scene and the seriousness of the situation as well as understanding the need for additional help and the risks to the rescuer's personal safety are all drummed into the heads of emergency professionals. While there are many things that should be reserved just for the professionals, assessing a situation is not one of them. From the moment you arrive at the scene of a traumatic or medical emergency, you'll need to mentally run through the assessment checklist shown on the opposite page. Committing this checklist to memory can help calm you during what might be a very chaotic scene and can lead to a better outcome for the patient.

The patient and scene assessment is broken into three parts (as shown to the right): the primary assessment, the ABCs and the secondary assessment. The primary assessment, which we'll review first, has six steps. In addition to explaining what should be accomplished with each step, I'll also present you with a scenario to put that primary assessment into practice. After completing the primary assessment, a rapid assessment of the patient's airway, breathing and circulation (ABC) will be conducted. I'll walk you through what to do if any of those are deficient. We'll wrap up this chapter by discussing what a rapid trauma assessment is and how you can use an "emergency move" to safely relocate an injured patient.

PATIENT AND SCENE ASSESSMENT

MEDICAL AND TRAUMATIC EMERGENCY CHECKLIST

Primary Assessment:

1. Determine scene safety.
2. Determine the need for additional resources, including calling 911 or dispatching someone to seek additional manpower.
3. Develop a general impression of the patient, such as whether you're dealing with a trauma or medical patient, whether he or she appears to be conscious or unconscious, etc. This general assessment can help you to take a mental pause to plot your course of action.
4. Determine the patient's mental status using the AVPU (Alert, Voice, Pain, Unresponsive) scale.
5. Assess and treat any immediate life threats, such as serious arterial bleeding, a compromised airway, a penetrating chest wound, etc.
6. For trauma patients, assess the need for spinal immobilization.

The ABCs:

- Assess the patient's AIRWAY. For a patient whose airway is blocked, open it using the head-tilt/chin-lift or the jaw-thrust method. Clear the airway of obstructions.
- Assess the patient's BREATHING rate and quality. For a patient with inadequate rate or volume of breath or who is not breathing, begin rescue breaths.
- Assess the patient's CIRCULATION, including pulse and color, temperature and condition of the skin. For a patient with no pulse, initiate access and use of an automatic external defibrillator (AED) and begin chest compressions.

Secondary Assessment:

- Conduct a Rapid Trauma Assessment to look for other life threats that you previously missed or for non-life threats, including DCAP-BTLS — deformities, contusions, abrasions, punctures/penetrations, burns, tenderness, lacerations or swelling.

1. Assess Scene Safety

Prior to entering any scene of a medical or traumatic emergency, you must first determine whether the scene is safe and secure or if it is a risk to you and other rescuers. If you run headlong into a situation that isn't safe, you risk becoming a victim yourself, making the job of subsequent rescuers even more difficult. For example, what risks might you want to account for if you came upon the scene on this page? If the victim is lying on a busy roadway, you should ensure that traffic has stopped before proceeding. Is the car still running and in gear? If so, place it in park, apply the emergency brake and remove the keys before proceeding. If you weren't a witness to what occurred, is there any other explanation for the victim lying in front of the car that could constitute a risk to you and other rescuers? For example, is it possible she was assaulted? If so, is the assailant still at the scene? While it might sound cruel, if you are not convinced that the scene is secure, you should not proceed until directed by the professionals.

Lastly, after you have determined that the scene is safe but *before* attending to the patient, you must ensure that you have your own personal protective equipment, which should *always* include nitrile gloves.

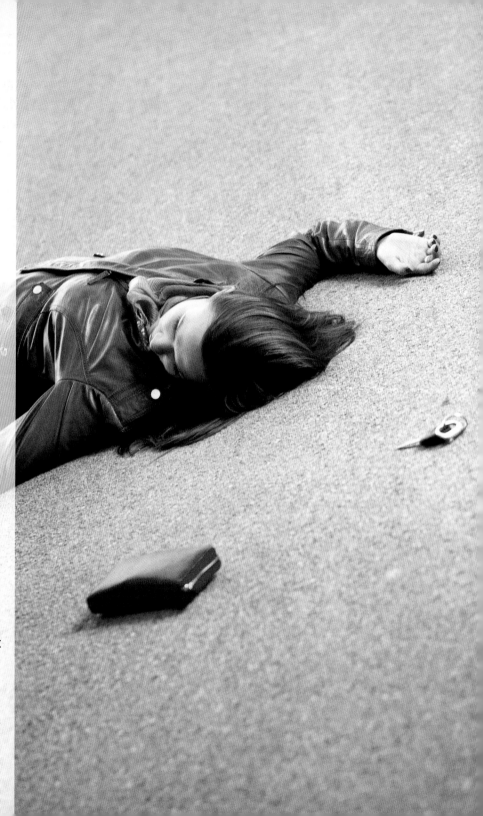

ASSESS SCENE SAFETY

The first action in our primary assessment is determining scene safety. Regardless of whether first responders were trained as police officers, firefighters, paramedics or EMTs, they all learn that the No. 1 responsibility is their own personal safety. That has to do with more than the police, fire and EMS departments wanting employees to make it home safe. It's because the risk to rescuers dramatically *increases* based upon the number of victims needing rescue. If a potential rescuer runs headlong into a situation that isn't safe, he or she risks becoming a victim. If the rescuer requires rescue, it puts subsequent rescuers at greater risk. As an example, let's say that an individual becomes trapped in the collapse of a ravine while hiking. As cruel as it may seem to not immediately jump to that person's rescue, if the walls of the ravine haven't been shored up, any rescuer jumping into action risks doubling or tripling the next rescuer's job *and* risk. Regardless of whether the traumatic or medical emergency you find yourself in is a violent attack in the middle of the city, a heart attack at the family cabin or a tumble off of a cliff miles from rescue, your overriding responsibility is to your *own personal safety*.

What's the first rule for rescuers? Don't become a victim yourself.

Safety for the Victim

Scene safety means more than just safety to the rescuers. It must also be a measurement of whether the scene constitutes a further risk to the patient, which may cause you to reorder priorities. For example, let's say that you come upon an accident where a pedestrian has been struck by a motor vehicle. If the vehicle is unstable and risks rolling over the patient, your first priority would be to remove the patient from further danger. That move would need to occur before treatment began on his or her injuries (and even before you have a chance to fully protect a possible spine injury). We'll talk about how to perform two emergency moves at the end of this chapter.

Personal Protective Equipment

When determining scene safety, fire, EMS and police personnel determine what type of personal protective equipment they need to get the job done as safely as possible. For firefighters, personal protective equipment (PPE) would include bunker gear, a helmet and boots, gloves, an air pack and mask, and other important items that weigh the firefighter down by 45-75 pounds. But for EMS and nonprofessional rescuers, the total weight of PPE required for most traumatic and medical emergencies can be measured in fractions of an ounce. Because of the number of blood-borne illnesses that can turn the rescuer into a victim (even if the diagnosis isn't until months later), wearing nitrile gloves anytime you're in contact with a patient is a *critically* important part of your protocol. Nitrile gloves not only help to protect the rescuer from potential harm but also protect the patient. Rescuers rarely have time to stop at the sink and scrub their hands for several minutes with hot water and surgical-grade soap before attending to the patient. Keep several pairs of nitrile gloves in your emergency first-aid kit, in your glove box or in your purse.

2. Determine the Need for Additional Resources

At this cardiac arrest scene, what additional resources are needed to help? This is the time to take a leadership role. Direct one bystander to retrieve an AED and another bystander to make a call to 911, providing him or her with specific information to relay to the dispatcher. Determine if you need additional bystanders to assist in the tasks of CPR or in moving the patient from any danger. Many treatments will have far more positive outcomes when the team involved is operating under the direction of a leader. For example, it's estimated that you must apply 100-125 pounds of pressure to a cardiac arrest patient's chest to achieve a proper depth of 2 inches. While that might be easy to perform in the classroom, it can become exhausting within minutes of a real event. At the scene shown on this page, rotating those tasks among two or more trained or semi-trained individuals can make the difference between life and death for this patient.

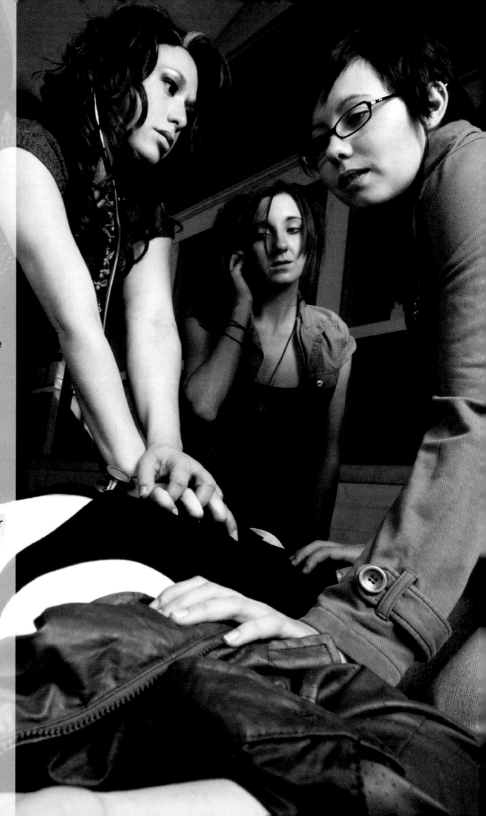

DETERMINE THE NEED FOR ADDITIONAL RESOURCES

The next step is to determine the need for additional resources. In any area with a telephone or cellphone coverage, your first priority is as simple as a phone call to 911. Do *not* delay this call for even a few minutes. Regardless of how well-trained you are, in the case of a serious traumatic or medical emergency, your patient's chances of survival depend upon how quickly EMS arrives at his or her side (and, in many cases, how quickly EMS delivers the patient to the emergency room). The sooner you can get EMS to your patient or your patient to EMS, the greater the chances of survival.

Also, additional resources could mean different things depending upon the emergency, your location and who might be available. You might simply need manpower to lift an injured patient or to lift something off of him or her. You might need one or two additional trained or semi-trained individuals to assist with and rotate the tasks of CPR. Or you might need to send a runner to find the closest AED. Step into the leadership role and delegate these tasks. As I mentioned in the preface, the most common response of bystanders during a medical or traumatic emergency after calling 911 is to do nothing. Don't be that person.

Your first priority is as simple as a phone call to 911. Do not delay this call for even a few minutes.

Evacuate or Shelter in Place?

As mentioned, part of getting access to additional resources is a call to 911. But in a case where you may find yourself outside of cellphone coverage and hours or days from EMS coverage, you'll need to make a determination on whether you should evacuate the patient or whether you should send someone to make contact with EMS while you shelter in place. There is no single right answer to that question, and many variables will come into play:

• Does evacuation risk exacerbating the patient's condition? For example, if the patient has broken ribs or a broken pelvis, any movement risks damaging underlying vessels or organs, and sheltering in place may be a better choice.

• Are there adequate resources to evacuate? While it might look easy on TV dramas and in the movies, it is actually far more difficult to move a patient than you might expect. That is especially true if the patient must be moved over rough terrain, in the dark or at altitude or if the patient is obese. Rescuers can quickly become exhausted before the patient has been fully evacuated, which might leave the patient in a new location far less conducive to EMS rescue than the original location. Unless you're confident that you have adequate resources to fully and safely evacuate the patient, you should elect to shelter in place with the patient and send one or more people to bring EMS to your patient.

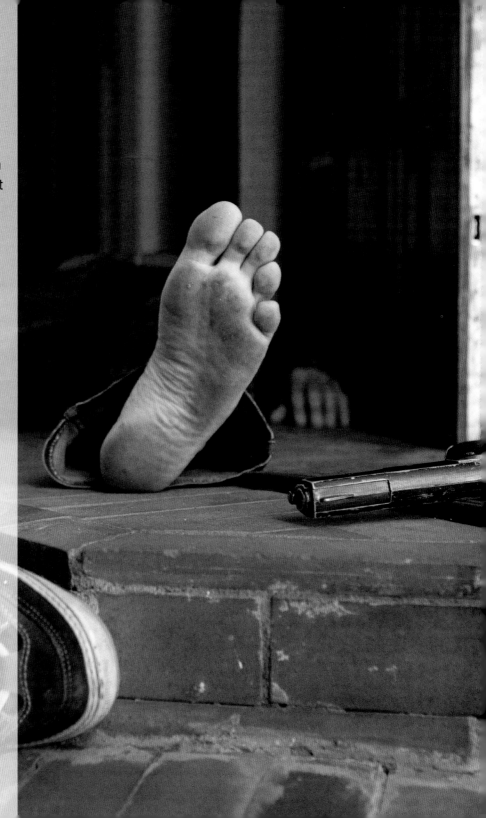

3. Develop a General Impression

When approaching the scene and the patient, gain a general impression of what you see. In the example on this page, does it appear that this is a victim of blunt trauma, a stabbing or a gunshot injury? Or could this be a medical emergency, such as cardiac arrest? Do you see any obvious life threats, such as spurting or pooling blood? What explanation could there be for why his shoe is off? What does the presence of the gun tell you, if anything? Is there an apparent mechanism of injury that would lead you to prepare for spinal immobilization?

4. Assess the Patient's Level of Awareness

Is the patient oriented to person, place, time and events? In other words, does he answer your questions and does he know who he is, where he is, when it is and what happened? If he does answer your questions, are his responses correct? If he doesn't respond verbally, does he respond to painful stimulus such as a pinch on the shoulder, a sternal rub or scraping an object on the bottom of his foot? Or is he completely unresponsive?

DEVELOP A GENERAL IMPRESSION OF THE PATIENT AND OF THE SITUATION

Though we have determined that the scene is safe and what additional resources we need, we're still not quite ready to jump in and begin treating the patient. We'll want to establish a general impression of the patient and the situation. This impression can be done from across the room to establish your next steps. Even before getting hands-on, you can attempt to determine: Is this a medical or traumatic event? Does the person appear to be alert? If so, how alert? Are there any obvious life threats, such as pooling or spurting blood? If it is a traumatic injury, does the mechanism of injury (MOI) seem to be serious enough that it could have caused spinal or head injuries? Taking a few seconds to perform this general assessment can help you to see the big picture and avoid the tunnel vision that can occur during these stressful situations.

Is This a Traumatic or a Medical Emergency?

While it might seem easy to determine if you're dealing with a traumatic or a medical emergency, sometimes there are unknown factors. For example, if you came upon a patient having a seizure, a "tunnel-vision" assumption would be that you're dealing with a medical emergency such as epilepsy. But taking a few seconds to see the big picture might make you also aware that the patient has a head injury. Did the seizure cause a fall that lead to the head injury? Or did a fall cause a head injury that lead to the seizure? If you came upon a patient who was in a low-speed car crash, a "tunnel-vision" assumption would be that you might

be dealing with some minor trauma. But taking a few seconds to see the big picture might make you also aware that the patient is unconscious, leading you to include the possibility that a medical condition (such as cardiac arrest or anaphylaxis) could have occurred first. Those few extra seconds could cause your mental gears to switch from, "I'm dealing with a minor car crash with minor injuries," to, "This could be a life-threatening medical emergency, and I will proceed with that assumption until proven otherwise."

ASSESS THE PATIENT'S LEVEL OF AWARENESS

Our next step is to determine our patient's level of awareness. Determining a patient's level of awareness can help you to determine the seriousness of the problem. If the patient is alert and aware, he or she will be your best source of information. For example, he or she might say, "I fell off the ladder!" or, "Pain is radiating down my left arm!" Use the AVPU scale below to determine the patient's awareness.

A - The patient is **ALERT** and oriented to self, time and place.

V - The patient responds to your **VERBAL** commands but does not answer appropriately or at all.

P - The patient only responds to **PAINFUL** stimulus, such as a shoulder pinch or sternal rub.

U - The patient is completely **UNRESPONSIVE**.

For any patient below "V," you should be prepared to maintain an open airway with the head-tilt/chin-lift or jaw-thrust methods discussed on Pages 34-35.

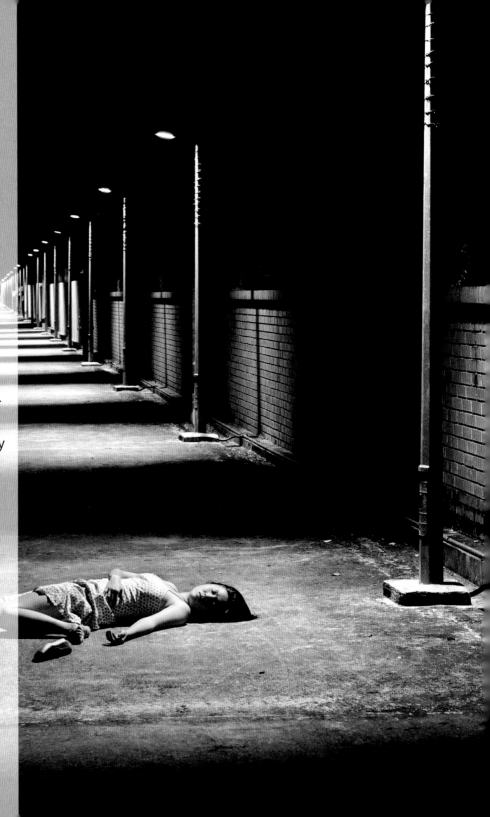

5. Assess and Treat Major Life Threats

Our first hands-on action will be to search the patient for and treat any major life threats. Life threats are traumatic injuries or medical conditions that are so serious that the patient risks death if the condition isn't corrected in minutes.

As you approach the patient in this scene, what immediate life threats would you search for? If this is an assault victim, she may be suffering from severe arterial bleeding, a penetrating wound to the torso or a serious abdominal injury. Scan the patient from head to toe, looking for pooling or spurting blood. Are any other life threats apparent, such as a lack of breathing or lack of pulse? Are there any signs or symptoms of life-threatening medical conditions, such as a diabetic emergency (moist, cool skin and an elevated heart rate) or an anaphylactic reaction (swelling of the skin, lips, tongue, hands or feet and the presence of hives)? If the patient has multiple traumatic injuries and you're not sure where to start, ask yourself, "What will kill my patient first?"

FIND AND TREAT MAJOR LIFE THREATS

Although it's taken a few pages to explain the assessment steps, it should take no more than 60 seconds in a real-life emergency. So our next step, a *critical* step, is to assess and treat any immediate life threats. Life threats are exactly that: deficiencies so significant that if not corrected immediately, they will result in the patient's rapid deterioration and death. Immediate life threats can include:

- Serious arterial bleeding, characterized by bright red, spurting blood
- An airway blocked by blood, vomit, teeth, the tongue, food or other object
- A stopped heart
- A penetrating chest wound, broken ribs or a serious abdominal injury
- A broken femur or pelvis, which bleed heavily and can cause the patient to lose as much as a third of his or her blood volume
- Severe allergic reactions (referred to as anaphylaxis)
- Diabetic emergencies, which can cause a patient to rapidly deteriorate

The great news is we'll be addressing each of these and other life threats in Chapters 2 and 3.

When dealing with a patient who is suffering from multiple traumatic injuries, you may not know where to start. The question you must ask yourself is, "What will kill my patient first?" The answer to that will set you on the right path.

Distracting Injuries

As you're evaluating the victim for significant life threats, don't be distracted by what are appropriately called "distracting injuries." These are injuries that might be very obvious and give the *appearance* of being serious life threats, drawing our attention away from more serious deficiencies. Two common distracting injuries are cuts to the scalp and "road rash." The scalp is rich with capillaries and will bleed profusely if cut (but rarely enough to cause anything more than a gag reflex in bystanders). Road rash (such as what might occur if a motorcyclist drops his or her bike and skids along the asphalt) might *appear* like a significant injury, but it doesn't rise to the level of a life threat. Focusing on those injuries might distract the rescuer for critical minutes while more-serious injuries (such as a knife wound to the chest or a broken femur) go undetected and drain the life from the patient

After any serious trauma, the adrenaline and endorphins coursing through your patient may mask the pain of serious injuries, and the patient may not even realize that he or she has been seriously injured. To find major life threats, do a head-to-toe search. When dealing with a patient who is suffering from multiple traumatic injuries, you may not know where to start. The question you must ask yourself is, "What will kill my patient first?" The answer to that will set you on the right path.

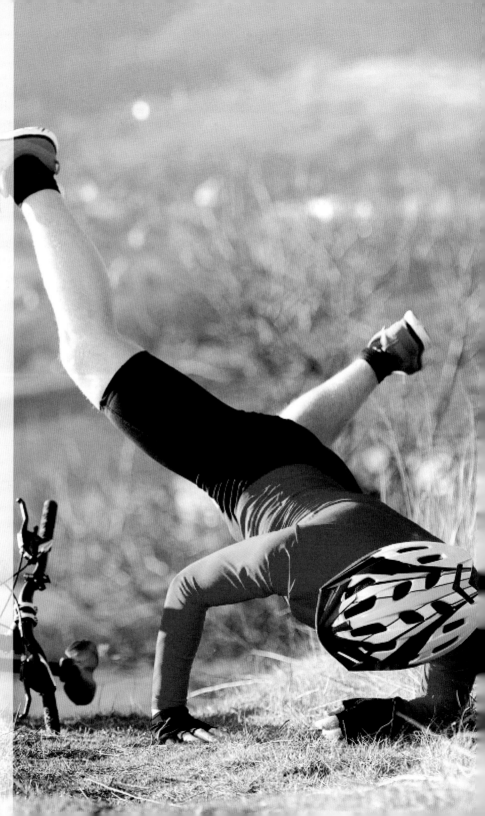

6. Determine the Need for Spinal Immobilization

It's easy to make the assumption that spinal precautions should be taken when a passenger is ejected from a car crash. Too often, though, those same precautions are not being taken for other more common accidents, such as falls or bicycle accidents or after soccer players' heads collide. If you came upon this patient who was thrown from his bike, how would you assess whether spinal precautions should be taken? How would your opinion change if witnesses reported that the patient had momentarily lost consciousness or if the patient was complaining of significant neck pain when moving his head from side to side? If the patient is up and moving around, it may be a difficult decision to ask him to lie down so that you can take precautions. If you believe that the MOI was serious enough to warrant those precautions (or if one or more of the additional risk conditions exist), taking those precautions may protect the patient from significant and *permanent* injury to the spinal cord.

DETERMINE THE NEED FOR SPINAL IMMOBILIZATION

Next, we're going to determine whether a head or spinal injury may have occurred, which would indicate that we should take additional precautions. Paramedics, EMTs and other first responders are trained to assess what's called the "mechanism of injury" (MOI), or what caused the injury to a trauma patient, in order to determine whether spinal immobilization is warranted. The more serious the MOI, the more likely a spinal injury may have occurred, requiring precautions to avoid further damaging the spinal cord. While common sense is going to play a part in a decision to implement spinal immobilization, some MOIs are so significant that an assumption should be made that a spinal injury is probable until proven otherwise. Examples of those MOIs include:

- Any direct blow to the head or neck, which would include a significant punch or being hit with a blunt object. An example would be a sport injury where players' heads collide.
- Any diving incident where the individual struck his head.
- Any fall from greater than a standing height or *any* height for patients older than 65.
- An ejection from a motorized or human-powered machine, such as being thrown from a bicycle.
- Any automobile accident where another occupant of the vehicle was killed. This is obviously an indication that the forces applied to the vehicle were significant, and we should assume the other occupant of the vehicle may have head or spinal injuries until proven otherwise.

- Lastly, in any automobile accident where there is more than 12 inches of intrusion into the passenger space, the vehicle has rolled over or airbags have deployed, we should be aware that spinal injuries may have occurred.

Additional Risk Factors for Trauma Patients

In addition, if any of the following occur, the rescuers should take spinal immobilization precautions:

- If the patient is not alert to person, place, time and events. To test this, you can simply ask the individual if he knows his name, where he is, if he knows what the date is and another simple fact, such as who the president of the United States is.
- When a loss of consciousness has occurred. Back to my example of two soccer players colliding, if one of those players lost consciousness for even a moment, you should *not* allow that player to get up and walk around.
- Those same precautions should also be taken if the individual has any pain or tenderness upon gently touching the spine.
- If you can't detect a pulse in one or more extremity, if the patient can't feel you touching the fingers or toes on one or more extremity, or if the patient can't move the fingers or toes on one or more extremity, those symptoms could indicate a spinal injury.
- If the patient feels significant pain upon moving his or her head from side to side or forward and backward, err on the side of caution and perform the simple procedure I'll explain on Page 33.

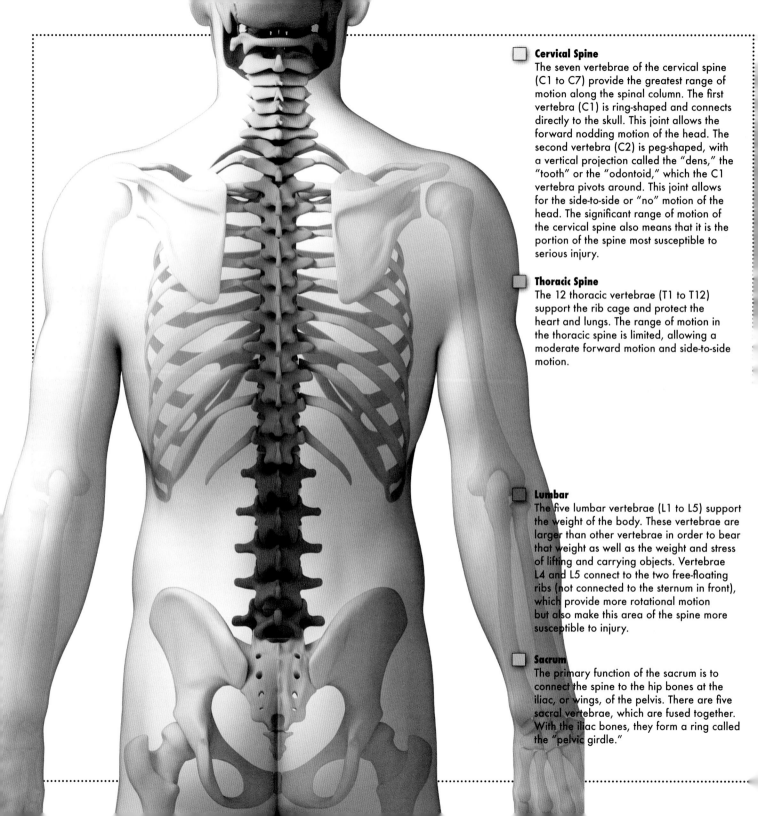

Cervical Spine

The seven vertebrae of the cervical spine (C1 to C7) provide the greatest range of motion along the spinal column. The first vertebra (C1) is ring-shaped and connects directly to the skull. This joint allows the forward nodding motion of the head. The second vertebra (C2) is peg-shaped, with a vertical projection called the "dens," the "tooth" or the "odontoid," which the C1 vertebra pivots around. This joint allows for the side-to-side or "no" motion of the head. The significant range of motion of the cervical spine also means that it is the portion of the spine most susceptible to serious injury.

Thoracic Spine

The 12 thoracic vertebrae (T1 to T12) support the rib cage and protect the heart and lungs. The range of motion in the thoracic spine is limited, allowing a moderate forward motion and side-to-side motion.

Lumbar

The five lumbar vertebrae (L1 to L5) support the weight of the body. These vertebrae are larger than other vertebrae in order to bear that weight as well as the weight and stress of lifting and carrying objects. Vertebrae L4 and L5 connect to the two free-floating ribs (not connected to the sternum in front), which provide more rotational motion but also make this area of the spine more susceptible to injury.

Sacrum

The primary function of the sacrum is to connect the spine to the hip bones at the iliac, or wings, of the pelvis. There are five sacral vertebrae, which are fused together. With the iliac bones, they form a ring called the "pelvic girdle."

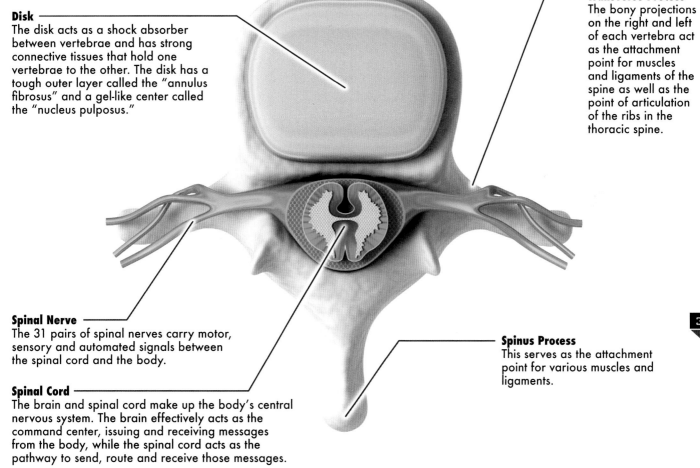

Disk
The disk acts as a shock absorber between vertebrae and has strong connective tissues that hold one vertebrae to the other. The disk has a tough outer layer called the "annulus fibrosus" and a gel-like center called the "nucleus pulposus."

Transverse Process
The bony projections on the right and left of each vertebra act as the attachment point for muscles and ligaments of the spine as well as the point of articulation of the ribs in the thoracic spine.

Spinal Nerve
The 31 pairs of spinal nerves carry motor, sensory and automated signals between the spinal cord and the body.

Spinal Cord
The brain and spinal cord make up the body's central nervous system. The brain effectively acts as the command center, issuing and receiving messages from the body, while the spinal cord acts as the pathway to send, route and receive those messages.

Spinus Process
This serves as the attachment point for various muscles and ligaments.

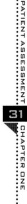

SPINAL INJURIES
PROVIDING MANUAL STABILIZATION

Paramedics, EMTs and other first responders are taught to quickly evaluate a traumatic situation to determine if the MOI was significant enough to cause spinal injuries, therefore requiring spinal immobilization. Regardless of the seriousness of the MOI, you'll also need to look for other indicators, such as whether the patient has a deficiency in circulation, motor function or sensory functions in any extremity. This means that if your patient

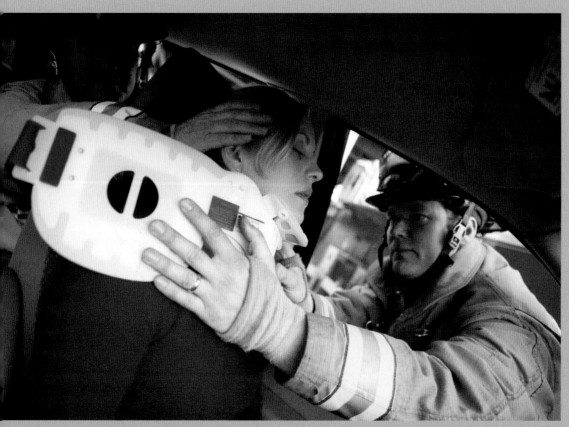

lacks a pulse in any extremity, is unable to move his or her fingers or toes, or is unable to feel your touch on any extremity, spinal immobilization should occur. In the photo on this page, the firefighters are placing a C-collar on the patient ("C" refers to the cervical spine), but also notice that the firefighter in the backseat is providing manual stabilization to the patient's spine by simply holding her head in place. This manual stabilization can be done in any situation where a spinal injury is suspected. If EMS is hours or days away, you should further stabilize your patient's head and neck with rolled towels on either side of his or her head (taped in place) or by using the field-expedient cervical collar demonstrated in Chapter 2 (using a SAM splint).

Taking Manual Stabilization

So let's talk about what kind of spinal precautions you can take, even if EMS is on its way to the scene. While EMS may apply a collar (referred to as "C-collar" due to the cervical spine it protects) and package the patient up on a backboard — complete with blocks holding the patient's head in place — your precautions can be much simpler. Immobilization at this stage of the process can be limited to one rescuer manually stabilizing the patient's head, holding it in-line with the rest of the spine, while a second rescuer continues with the assessment. If you are a single rescuer, do *not* delay the remainder of the assessment — in particular, don't delay an assessment of your patient's ABCs while attempting to stabilize the spine. After the assessment is completed, full spinal immobilization of the patient can occur. I'll add, once you have taken in-line spinal stabilization, do *not* release it for any reason until EMS or another rescuer has taken over.

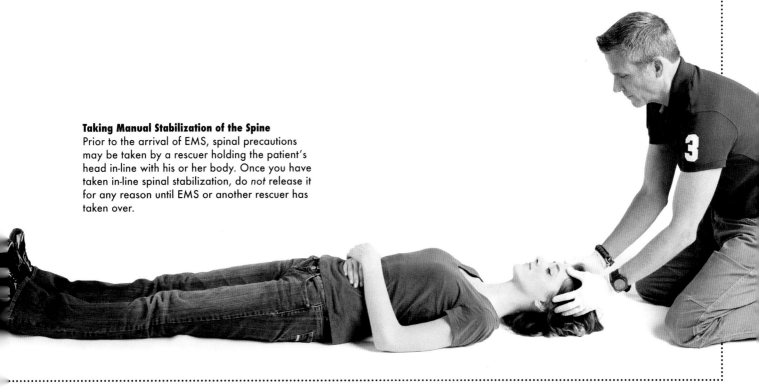

Taking Manual Stabilization of the Spine
Prior to the arrival of EMS, spinal precautions may be taken by a rescuer holding the patient's head in-line with his or her body. Once you have taken in-line spinal stabilization, do *not* release it for any reason until EMS or another rescuer has taken over.

ASSESS THE ABCS

Our next major step is to assess the patient's ABCs: Airway, Breathing and Circulation.

A: Assessing the Patient's Airway

Aside from starting with the first letter of the alphabet, the airway falls first in the list because everything that we're doing to save the life of a critically injured or ill patient has to do with whether or not the brain is receiving ample oxygen. Even if the patient's heart is continuing to beat, if we don't have an open airway, we really have nothing. For conscious patients, the simplest method of determining whether the airway is patent, or open, is to ask the patient what the problem is. If he or she responds with something like,

PATENT
[**pah**-tunt]
Open, unobstructed, not closed.

"I fell off that cliff!," you can conclude that the airway is open and move on to the next step in the assessment. If your patient is unconscious or has an altered level of consciousness, you'll need to look, listen and feel. Place your ear to the patient's mouth, watch for the chest to rise, listen for breathing and feel for his or her breath on your ear. If you *do* hear or feel breathing and see the chest rise, you can move on to "B." If you *don't* see, hear or feel breathing, you'll need to open the patient's airway. Although professionals might eventually turn to a King Airway or an endotracheal tube, they'll start with the head-tilt/chin-lift or the jaw-thrust technique (as shown on the opposite page).

Clearing the Airway of Blockages

If the patient does not begin breathing after you have opened his or her airway, you must check to determine if the airway is blocked by food, vomit, broken teeth, blood or another object. If you discover a blockage, it must be removed. To do so, roll the patient on his or her side. If another rescuer is maintaining in-line stabilization of the head due to a suspected spinal injury, that rescuer must maintain stabilization during the roll and should call out the command: "Roll on one, two, three." After the patient is on his or her side, sweep the mouth with a gloved finger from one side of the mouth to the other. Only insert your finger as far as you can see, and never do a "blind sweep" where you risk pushing the blockage deeper into the airway. After clearing the blockage to the best of your ability, return the patient to his or her back, coordinating the move with other rescuers, and reopen the airway using the head-tilt/chin-lift or the jaw-thrust technique.

As a side note, if the thought of inserting your finger into a stranger's mouth to remove food, vomit, broken teeth or blood is distasteful, remember that the first item in your personal emergency first-aid kit should be several pairs of nitrile gloves.

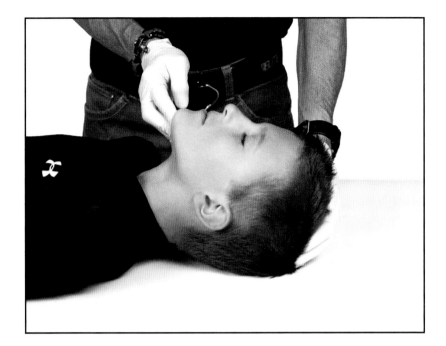

Head Tilt/Chin Lift

For patients who *do not* have a suspected spinal injury, the airway can usually be opened by pressing down on the forehead and lifting the chin. This typically clears the tongue from the airway, which is the usual suspect in an airway blockage of an unconscious patient. As long as the patient is unconscious or has an altered mental status, you'll need to continue to hold this position to ensure the airway remains open.

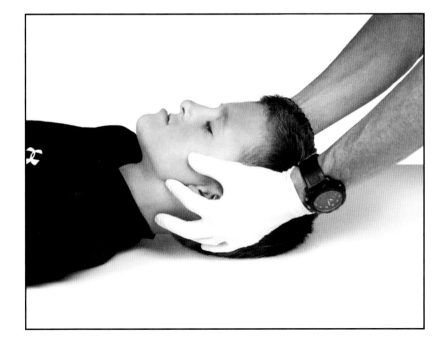

Jaw Thrust

For patients who *do* have a suspected spinal injury, the tongue can usually be cleared from the airway by pushing up from both sides of the jaw, forcing it upward (toward the ceiling). This can best be done if the rescuer positions himself or herself at the patient's head, facing the patient's feet. By forcing the jaw up, the tongue is lifted, clearing the airway without compromising the patient's spinal cord.

This is a more difficult position to hold and will typically require a second rescuer if rescue breaths must be delivered.

B: Assessing the Patient's Breathing Volume and Rate

You may assume that if the airway is clear, the patient must be getting adequate oxygen, but that's not always going to be the case. When assessing a patient's breathing, two factors matter, and *both* must be true for you to conclude that your patient's breathing is adequate.

Breathing Volume

First, your patient's tidal volume (the actual amount of air that he or she breathes in) must be adequate to draw fresh air down to the base of the lungs, which are rich in alveoli. Alveoli are responsible for the exchange of gases between the lungs and the blood in the capillaries. Even if your patient is breathing, if those breaths are extremely shallow (the volume is too low), your patient may still be starved of oxygen, and death will result unless you intervene.

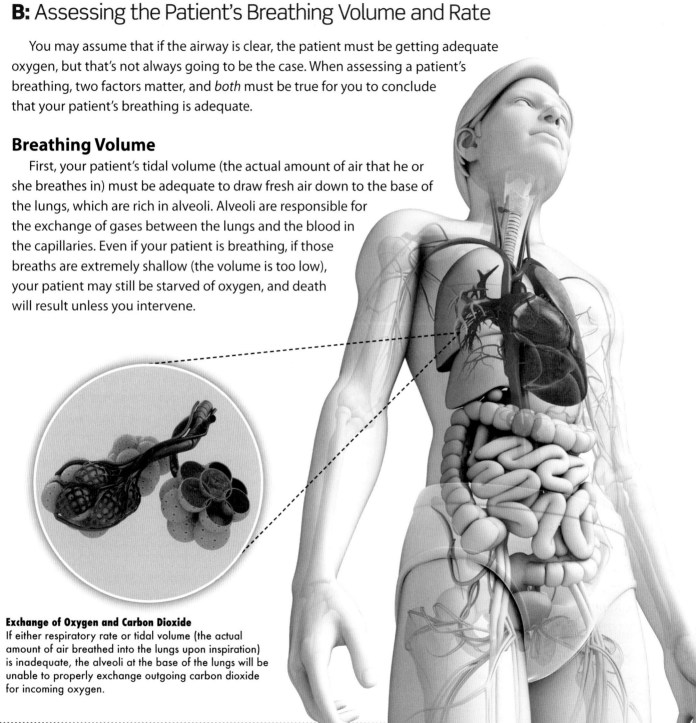

Exchange of Oxygen and Carbon Dioxide
If either respiratory rate or tidal volume (the actual amount of air breathed into the lungs upon inspiration) is inadequate, the alveoli at the base of the lungs will be unable to properly exchange outgoing carbon dioxide for incoming oxygen.

Breathing Rate

Second, your patient's rate of breathing (breaths per minute) must be appropriate to sustain his or her life. The normal breathing rate for a healthy adult is about 12-20 breaths per minute, while infants, toddlers and preschool children will have a normal rate of about 20-30 breaths per minute. A rate too *slow* can starve your patient of necessary oxygen. And a rate too *high* can cause the volume to be too low, since the lungs won't have time to fill completely. This will also result in the patient blowing off too much carbon dioxide, which must remain in proper balance for the respiratory system to work correctly.

Signs and Symptoms of Difficultly Breathing (Dyspnea)

- A rate that is too fast or too slow when compared to what is normal for the patient or what is normal for his or her age.
- Poor tidal volume, which can be indicated by an inadequate chest rise.
- Nasal flaring, which can indicate that the patient is making a significant effort to breathe.
- Retractions of the skin between or below the ribs or above the clavicles. These signs indicate that the patient is using accessory muscles to breathe, which shows that breathing takes tremendous effort. This will quickly exhaust the patient, leading to respiratory arrest, or apnea.

DYSPNEA
[dis-p-**knee**-a]
Breathing that is labored or difficult.

- Patient sitting in the tripod position with the elbows resting on the knees and leaning forward to reduce the breathing effort (referred to as "tripoding").
- Cyanosis, which I'll describe on Page 42.

APNEA
[**app**-knee-a]
A complete absence of breathing; respiratory arrest.

For any patient with an altered mental status who has inadequate rate or volume or who isn't breathing at all, you must begin rescue breaths at a rate of 10-12 breaths per minute using the procedure on the next page.

Rescue Breaths

If you're a bit squeamish about direct mouth-to-mouth contact, a must-have in your field first-aid kit is a pocket mask or a NuMask™.

Using a Pocket Mask

To properly use a pocket mask, you will perform the C/E method. Form your non-dominant hand into a "C" with your thumb and index finger, leaving your middle, ring and pinky fingers as an "E." You'll wrap the "C" around the mask to hold it in place and perform a head tilt/chin lift with the "E" by placing those three fingers directly on the bony part of the jaw. Don't sink those fingers into the soft tissue under the chin or you risk blocking the airway. As you deliver breaths at a rate of 10-12 per minute, which is one breath every five to six seconds, watch for the patient's chest to rise, which will indicate that you're performing rescue breaths properly. Since it does take practice to get a perfect seal with these masks, I suggest investing time in taking a Red Cross or American Heart Association CPR course, where you'll get a chance to put a pocket mask through its paces.

Using a NuMask

As mentioned, it can be difficult to get a perfect seal from a pocket mask, especially with patients who have bony faces, small chins or thick facial hair. A new mask gaining popularity actually isn't a mask at all. The NuMask operates more like a snorkel tube and uses a flexible mouthpiece placed *inside* the patient's mouth, between his or her lips and teeth (or gums if the patient happens to be missing teeth). Gaining a perfect seal with the NuMask is much simpler, even if the patient has dentures or is missing teeth. If there is a shortcoming to the NuMask, it's that it offers less of a barrier if the patient vomits during rescue breaths or CPR. I know that's not a pleasant picture, but it happens more often than not.

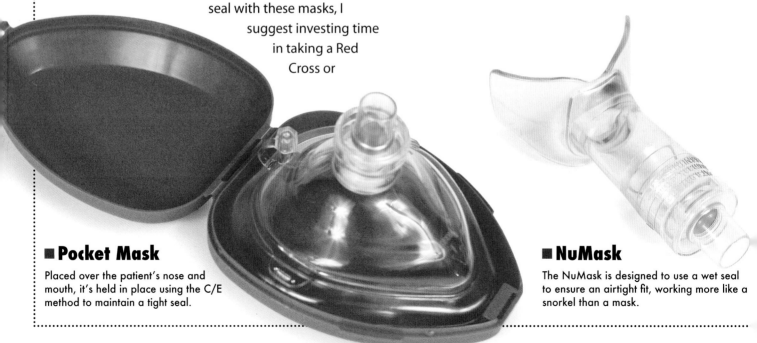

■ Pocket Mask
Placed over the patient's nose and mouth, it's held in place using the C/E method to maintain a tight seal.

■ NuMask
The NuMask is designed to use a wet seal to ensure an airtight fit, working more like a snorkel than a mask.

Step 1: Pocket Mask Setup

Form your non-dominant hand into a "C" with your thumb and index finger and an "E" with your middle, ring and pinky fingers.

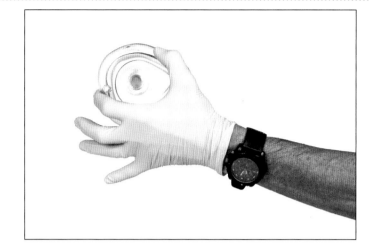

Step 2: Placing the Mask

Standing at the patient's head, hold the mask in place with the "C" and perform a head tilt/chin lift by placing those three "E" fingers directly on the bony part of the jaw. Don't sink those fingers into the soft tissue under the chin or you risk blocking the airway. As you deliver breaths at a rate of 10-12 per minute, which is one breath every five to six seconds, watch for the patient's chest to rise, indicating that you're performing rescue breaths properly.

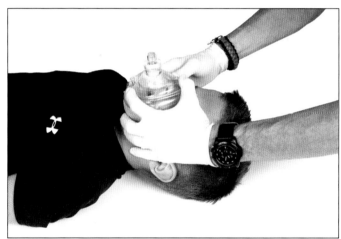

Using a NuMask

Slide the NuMask mouthpiece into the patient's mouth, between the lips and teeth or gums, similar to how you'd place a snorkel tube in your own mouth. Perform a standard head tilt/chin lift or jaw thrust and deliver breaths. Because the nose is not covered by the NuMask, the rescuer should pinch the patient's nose while delivering rescue breaths.

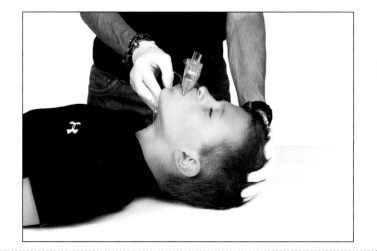

C: Assessing the Patient's Circulation

As mentioned, severe bleeding can quickly compromise a patient's cardiac system, leading to compensatory and decompensatory shock within minutes. This isn't caused by the actual blood loss. Instead, it's caused by the lack of oxygen to the brain since blood is the transport system responsible for delivering that oxygen. If that transport system is interrupted by blood loss because of the heart stopping or any other reason, the situation must be corrected within minutes or the patient risks death.

Serious external bleeding is an easy deficiency to notice (and we'll cover in Chapter 2 how to deal with it), but how would you determine if any other part of your patient's circulatory system was deficient? Checking for a pulse is a good first step. (As mentioned under "Airway," though, if your patient is talking to you, then you can also assume that his or her heart is still beating.) If your patient is unresponsive, you can assess the circulatory system by checking the patient's radial pulse, which is the pulse located in the wrist.

Feeling for a pulse is relatively simple. Apply pressure with the fingertips of your index and middle fingers directly on top of the hard tendons beneath the wrist. Then, slide those fingers into the indentation next to those tendons. While it might take some practice on friends or family, you'll be able to find a pulse within seconds using this method. If you're unable to find a radial pulse, the next step would be to check the patient's carotid pulse, located on the carotid arteries of the neck. To check for this pulse, you'll slide your two fingertips down the hard trachea until they fall into the indentation next to the trachea. This is typically a very easy pulse to find. If you're finding no pulse in an unresponsive patient, he or she is in cardiac arrest. You'll need to begin the chain of survival we will discuss in Chapter 3.

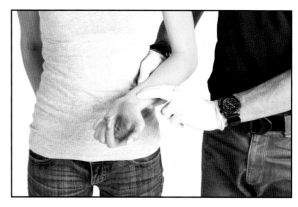

Finding a Radial Pulse
Apply pressure with the fingertips of your index and middle fingers directly on top of the hard tendons beneath the wrist, and then slide those fingers into the indentation next to those tendons. Count the number of beats for 15 seconds, and then multiply by four to find the heart rate in beats per minute.

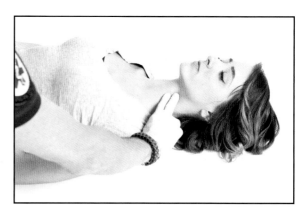

Finding a Carotid Pulse
Slide your two fingertips down the hard trachea until they fall into the indentation next to the trachea. Do not search for a pulse for more than 10 seconds, or you risk delaying lifesaving CPR.

NORMAL VITAL SIGNS					
	AGE	RESPIRATORY RATE	PULSE RATE	SYSTOLIC	DIASTOLIC
Newborn	Birth - 6 Weeks	30 - 50	120 - 160	74 - 100	50 - 68
Infant	7 Weeks - 1 Year	20 - 30	80 - 140	84 - 106	56 - 70
Toddler	1 - 2 Years	20 - 30	90 - 130	98 - 106	50 - 70
Preschool	2 - 6 Years	20 - 30	80 - 120	98 - 112	64 - 70
School Age	6 - 13 Years	18 - 30	(60 - 80) - 100	104 - 124	64 - 80
Adolescent	13 - 16 Years	(12 - 20) - 30	60 - 100	118 - 132	70 - 82
Adult	> 16 Years	12 - 20	60 - 100	100 - 150	60 - 90

Normal Vitals

While you wouldn't be expected to memorize what normal vital signs should be for patients of different ages, the table on this page will give you a good indication of what normal *might* be, at least for a patient of your own age or for your spouse and children.

For example, in a healthy 50-year-old male, I would expect to find his resting heart rate to fall somewhere between 60 and 100 beats per minute, as shown on the table above. But if that same individual had just finished working out or running a few miles, I wouldn't be surprised to find his heart rate up around 120 or even higher. On the other hand, if I found that heart rate in a patient who had passed out in a restaurant, it would be considered abnormal, leading me to believe there was a serious medical issue.

While checking a heart rate requires a tactile observation, respiratory rate — the rate at which the patient is breathing — is assessed simply by a visual observation. Without even comparing a patient's actual rate to the table above, it's fairly easy to conclude whether a patient is breathing too fast or too slow, both of which can indicate a problem.

'Reading' the Patient

EMS professionals will measure the status of a patient's circulatory and other systems by using a few diagnostic tools. These will include measuring the patient's heart rate, blood pressure and the percentage of saturated oxygen in the patient's blood (pulse oximetry) and even taking a snapshot of the electrical signals coursing through the patient's heart. But beyond all that, EMS personnel are also taught to "read" the patient. That means regardless of what the patient's blood pressure is or what the pulse oximetry reads, if the patient doesn't look right, decisions will be made based upon that information.

Some things that you can use to read your patient without diagnostic tools include:

Skin Condition

In this case, I'm not talking about looking for cuts, scrapes or contusions. I'm talking about checking if the patient's skin is moist or dry, if it has proper coloring versus being flushed or pale, and if it feels like it has the proper temperature versus feeling hot or cool and clammy. Pale, cool, clammy skin can indicate blood loss (which could be internal or external) and should be a warning sign that the patient is in or approaching shock. Hot, dry skin may indicate dehydration or heat stroke. EMS will also conduct a simple test by pressing a finger or two on the skin of the patient's arm. If the patient has adequate "perfusion" (the patient has adequate blood volume and blood pressure, and the blood has adequate oxygen), color should return to the spot that was pressed within two seconds. If it takes longer than that for color to return, you should prepare to treat your patient for shock. A significant perfusion problem would be immediately apparent if the patient's lips or nail beds were showing a bluish tinge, which is referred to as "cyanosis."

CYANOSIS

[sigh-uh-**noh**-sis]

A bluish discoloration of the skin and mucous membranes caused by a lack of oxygen in the blood.

Estimating Blood Pressure

You wouldn't normally need to concern yourself with knowing a patient's blood pressure if EMS were minutes away. In cases where EMS may be much farther out, however, estimating a patient's blood pressure can help you determine if something more serious, such as shock, is occurring.

You can estimate your patient's blood pressure while checking his or her pulse, as discussed earlier. If you are able to feel a pulse in your patient's wrist (the radial pulse), you can assume that his or her systolic blood pressure (the upper number) is at least around 80.

Cyanosis
A significant perfusion problem would be immediately apparent if your patient's lips or nail beds were showing a bluish tinge, which is referred to as "cyanosis." Cyanosis is usually accompanied by skin that is pale, cool and clammy.

The actual systolic blood pressure might be much higher than that, but the fact that you are able to feel the radial pulse indicates that it should be at least 80 and that pressure remains in your patient's blood vessels. If the radial pulse is missing but you are able to detect a femoral pulse (the pulse in the groin), you can estimate that the systolic blood pressure is at least 70. If the radial and femoral pulses are missing but you are able to detect a pulse in the carotid artery at the neck, your patient's systolic blood pressure is most likely not above 60.

Whenever your patient's radial pulses are absent, aggressive action should be taken to protect your patient from shock. Of course, if *no* pulses are present, you'll need to immediately begin CPR to artificially move oxygenated blood through your patient's system, and you'll need to get access to an AED. More on both of those topics in Chapter 3.

On that note, we have now completed the majority of our assessment. If done correctly, we have accounted for and corrected the most serious deficiencies in our patient. Though it was several pages of steps, in a real-life situation, even nonprofessionals can accomplish those tasks in five minutes or less. The reality is, you'll *need* to complete them in five minutes or less during a critical incident, such as a traumatic injury where serious bleeding is occurring.

At four to five minutes with no oxygenated blood, the body is at risk of crossing from compensatory shock (the body's systems try to compensate for a loss of blood pressure) to decompensatory shock (the body's systems begin to fail) to irreversible shock, when the only outcome is death.

The tasks you've accomplished so far are all you'll usually need to consider if EMS is arriving on scene or is just minutes away. On the other hand, if EMS is hours or days away, you'll need to continue with what's referred to as a "rapid trauma assessment" or "secondary assessment" to look for additional life threats as well as secondary (but non-life-threatening) injuries.

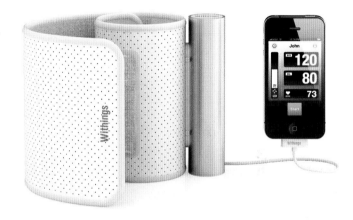

Smartphone-Compatible Blood Pressure Cuff

While not a requirement, if you'd like to take your patient assessment one step further, tens of thousands of people now monitor their own blood pressure at home using devices such as the Wireless Blood Pressure Monitor from Withings. Simply apply it to your patient's upper arm and initiate the cuff on your smartphone and you'll quickly have additional insight into your patient's current condition. Remember, however, regardless of what the blood pressure results are, you must also "read" your patient.

SECONDARY ASSESSMENT

A secondary assessment, or rapid trauma assessment, is a methodical, head-to-toe search to look for additional trauma, including life threats and non-life threats. For young children, you can reverse the search from toe to head to reduce anxiety. During this search, clothing can hide not only minor injuries that need treatment but also other serious life threats that haven't yet become apparent. On an ambulance, it's second nature for me to pull out my trauma shears and cut away jackets, shirts, boots, pants or anything else that's blocking my ability to properly perform a head-to-toe assessment.

Again, if EMS is minutes instead of an hour or more away and you're not concerned about any further life threats, leave the secondary assessment to the pros. If you find yourself in a situation where you believe it's necessary to perform a rapid trauma assessment, you'll need to expose your patient in as respectful a manner as possible. Of course, if the patient is conscious and able to answer your questions, you must explain what you're about to do and ask permission. If you find it necessary to perform this assessment, you'll be looking for additional life threats and what is referred to as DCAP-BTLS:

Deformities   **B**urns
Contusions   **T**enderness
Abrasions   **L**acerations
Penetrations   **S**welling

If you detect any of these injuries but it's *not* a life threat, simply note it and move on. Once the assessment is complete, you can decide what to do about the additional injury. As an example, if I'm performing

Neck
Look for a deviated trachea (shifted to one side or the other), which can indicate a tension pneumothorax.

Gently palpate the back of the neck to feel for any deformities to the spine.

Chest
Look and palpate for any deformities, penetrations or signs of other life-threatening injuries.

Abdomen
Look and palpate for any deformities, penetrations, evisceration or signs of other life-threatening injuries.

Head Trauma
Look and palpate (feel for) any obvious head injuries, including broken bones in the skull, eye sockets, nose and jaw. Look for blockages to the airway, such as vomit, blood or broken teeth. Look for clear fluid leaking from the ears, which is a sign of a basilar skull fracture.

Upper Extremities
Look and palpate for any deformities, and check for radial pulses in both arms.

Pupils
Determine if the patient's pupils are equal and if they react to light. If they are unequal, this may be a sign of a significant head injury.

a rapid trauma assessment on an unconscious motorcyclist who was struck by a car and is severely injured, I'm looking for other major life threats that I haven't previously found, such as uncontrolled bleeding. If I found that injury, I'd treat it using the technique we'll discuss in Chapter 2. On the other hand, if I discover that the lower arm is broken, I'll simply note it and move on. Once the assessment is done, I can decide whether I'll splint that injury or let the emergency room deal with it.

When performing a rapid trauma assessment, it's easiest to think of the body as a series of separate systems that you'll inspect individually. These systems are the head and neck, the chest, the abdomen, the pelvis, the upper extremities, the lower extremities and the back. When assessing each of these systems, you

PALPATE
[**pal**-pate]
To examine by touch, especially for the purpose of diagnosing disease or illness.

should look and palpate for DCAP-BTLS and life threats as demonstrated in the example below.

Pelvis
Look and gently palpate for any instability, which can indicate a broken pelvis. If a broken pelvis is discovered, treat it as a major life threat.

Lower Extremities
Look and palpate for any deformities, and check for pedal pulses in both feet. If a broken femur is discovered, treat it as a major life threat.

Back
With the assistance of other rescuers, log roll the patient to look for previously undetected bleeding. Also, palpate the spine to feel for any deformities.

EMERGENCY MOVES

We're going to end this chapter by discussing what should occur if you find it necessary to move an injured patient. In most cases, you will perform the primary assessment, including evaluating the patient's ABCs and addressing any immediate life threats before ever *considering* moving the patient. If EMS is on the way, there is usually no reason at all to move a patient from his or her current location. But in some cases, moving a patient *first* may take priority. Those cases include:

1. Situations when there is an *immediate* environmental or scene danger, constituting a greater threat to the patient than his or her current medical or traumatic condition.
2. Situations when the patient's current position or location is blocking you from performing lifesaving care, such as opening his or her airway or performing CPR.

Environmental or Scene Dangers

Environmental or scene dangers can include things like:

- Fire or the danger of fire
- Exposure to hazardous materials
- Other hazards, such as uncontrolled traffic, extreme weather, landslides, a building collapse or a hostile crowd

In all cases, before running headlong into performing any kind of rescue, you must always make your own personal safety a priority. As discussed previously, you're not going to do the patient or additional rescuers any favors if you become a victim. When your safety has been confirmed and an emergency move is required, use one of the emergency methods on the next pages.

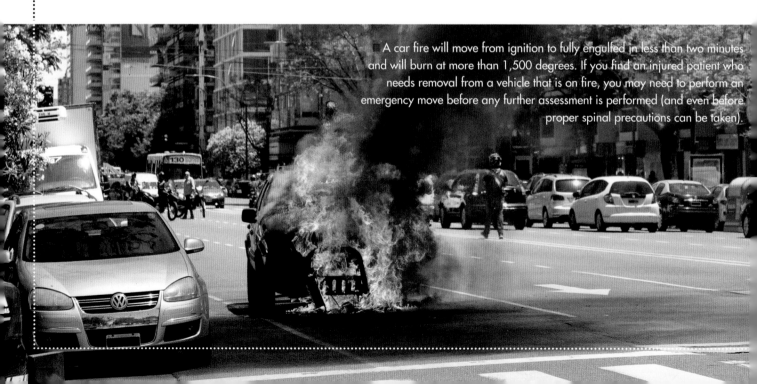

A car fire will move from ignition to fully engulfed in less than two minutes and will burn at more than 1,500 degrees. If you find an injured patient who needs removal from a vehicle that is on fire, you may need to perform an emergency move before any further assessment is performed (and even before proper spinal precautions can be taken).

■ Armpit Forearm Drag

To perform this move, roll your patient forward and then crouch behind him or her with your back straight. Reach your arms under his or her arms, locking your hands in front. In one smooth move, push up with your legs, keeping your back straight the entire time. Even with a patient much larger than you, you can support the weight as you shuffle backward. By cradling the patient's head against your body, you can minimize movement of the head and neck.

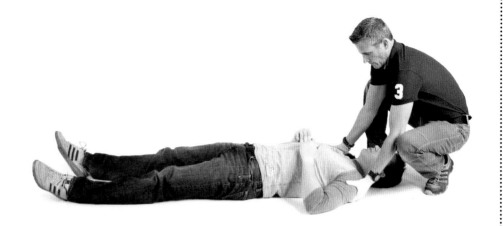

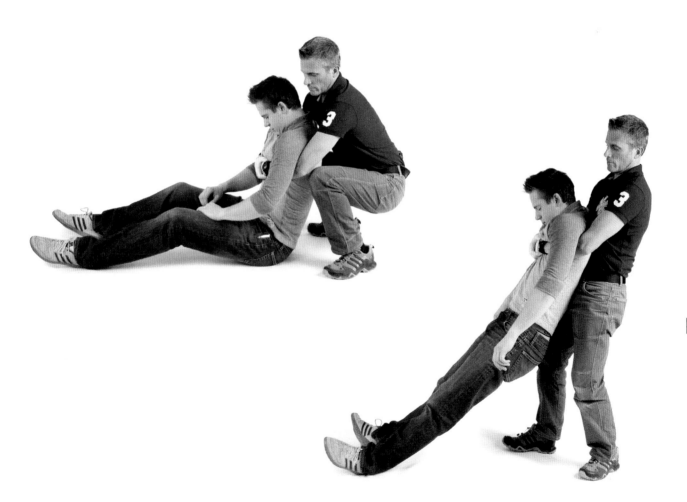

▪Shirt Drag

Like it sounds, the shirt drag is performed by grabbing the patient's shirt at the top (on one or both sides). This is a move that I might perform if there isn't room behind the patient for me to use the armpit forearm drag. Like the armpit forearm drag, it's important to lift with your legs rather than your back. During the shirt drag, you can cradle the patient's head against your forearms to minimize the movement of his or her head and neck.

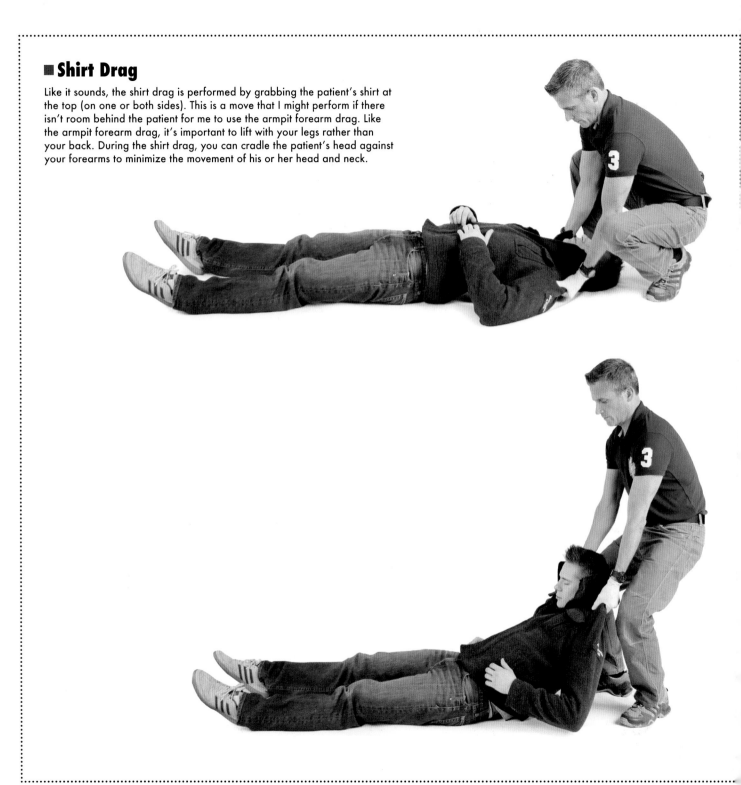

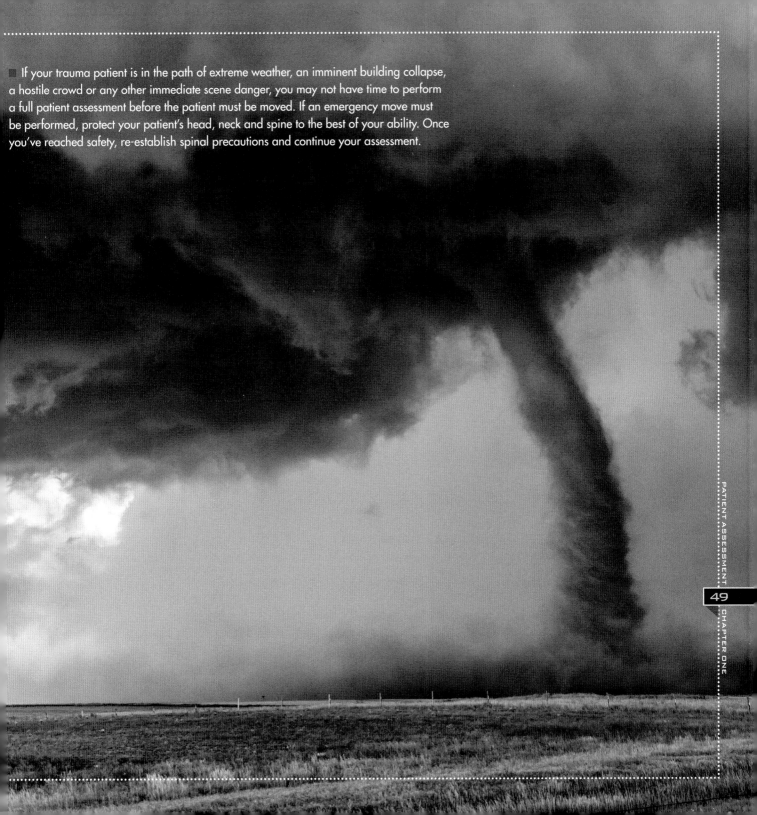

If your trauma patient is in the path of extreme weather, an imminent building collapse, a hostile crowd or any other immediate scene danger, you may not have time to perform a full patient assessment before the patient must be moved. If an emergency move must be performed, protect your patient's head, neck and spine to the best of your ability. Once you've reached safety, re-establish spinal precautions and continue your assessment.

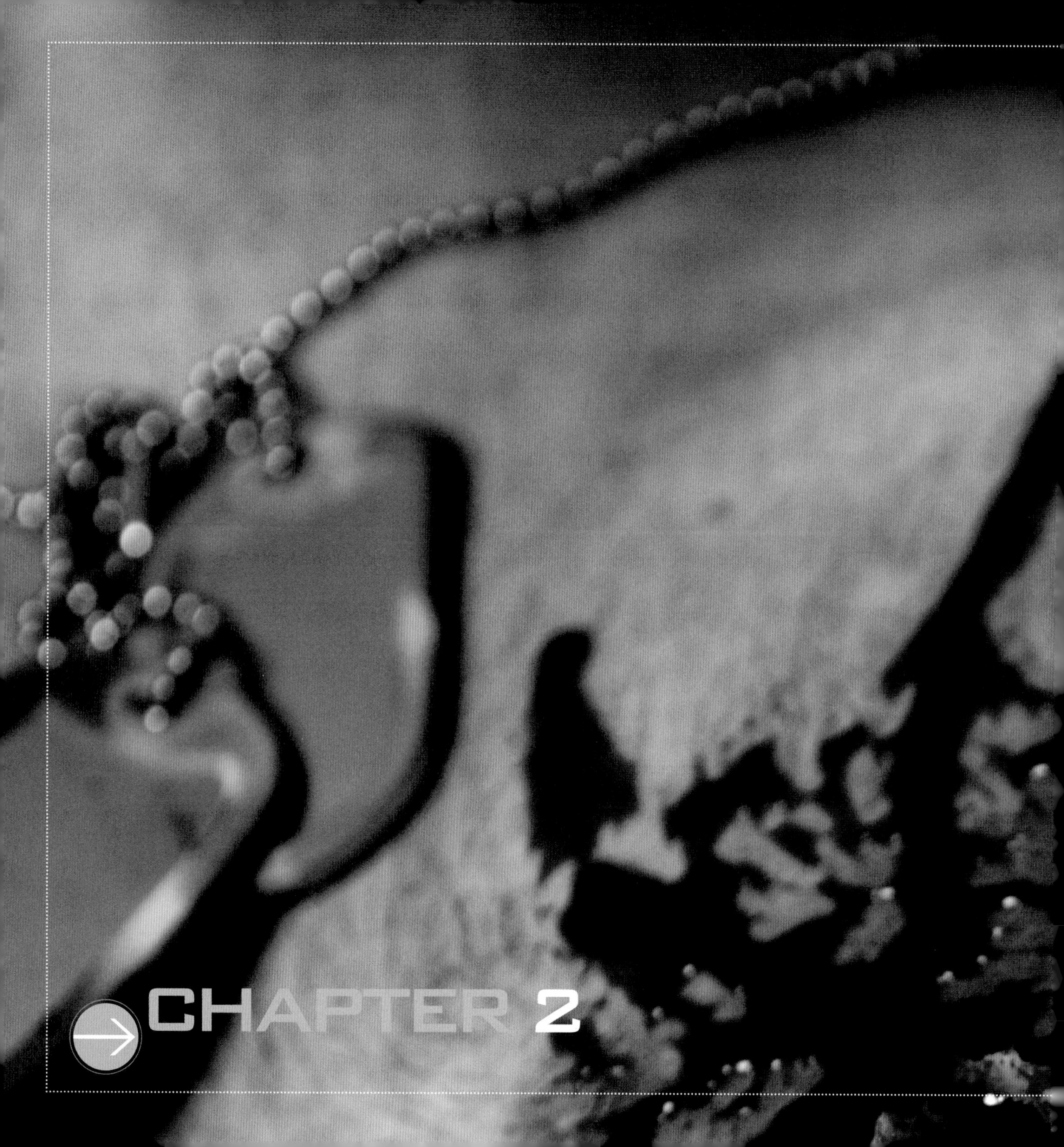

TRAUMATIC EMERGENCIES

- Severe Arterial Bleeding
- Maintenance of a Severe Laceration
- Penetrating Chest Injuries
- Severe Burns
- Musculoskeletal Trauma
- Femur Fractures
- Pelvis Fractures
- Rib Fractures and Flail Chest
- Head Trauma
- Trauma to the Eye

A severe traumatic injury can result from forces as everyday as a serious fall or automobile accident to forces as unthinkable as a shooting or stabbing as the result of an assault or robbery. This chapter will address the assessment and treatment of a number of trauma emergencies, including severe bleeding, a penetrating chest injury, flail chest, severe burns, musculoskeletal trauma (injury to the bones, muscles, ligaments or tendons) and trauma to the head and eye. It's fair to say that if a serious medical emergency (such as cardiac arrest or stroke) were to give the average nonprofessional anxiety, witnessing serious trauma will eclipse even that anxiety, meaning training and preparation are all the more important so that you can provide necessary, lifesaving care rather than freezing upon seeing spraying blood, a broken bone penetrating the skin or eviscerated internal organs. While the scene of a major medical emergency may have a number of bystanders who will increase the anxiety level, in serious trauma situations, the patient may actually increase that anxiety due to his or her appearance and screams. In such a chaotic situation, you must use the assessment checklist as explained in Chapter One to calm yourself, calm the patient and provide appropriate care to bridge the gap until EMS arrives on the scene. In this chapter, I'll not only cover the appropriate treatments for a number of traumatic

Slishman Traction Splint
While this might look like an everyday hiking pole or ski pole, it's actually a sophisticated traction splint, capable of dealing with a traumatic femur fracture in the field. You'll learn how to use this splint and even how to fashion a field-expedient substitute in this chapter.

conditions but also review a number of pieces of gear which should find their way into your own emergency first-aid kit, including a hemostatic dressing, such as QuikClot; a tourniquet, such as the CAT, the SOFTT-W or my new favorite, the Ratcheting Medical Tourniquet; a compression bandage, such as the "H" bandage or Israeli emergency bandage; a chest seal, such as the SAM or Bolin; and an eye shield, such as the H&H Combat Eye Shield. Since a wide variety of options exists for each of these product categories, I'll review the top products for each category and provide you with some of the pros and cons of each.

In this chapter, I'll also explain several more advanced interventions that might be required if you and your patient are hours or days away from EMS. Those advanced interventions include knowing how to hydraulically clean a serious laceration using a large bore syringe and sterilized water and how to use adhesive sutures, benzoin swabs and a gel bandage to close and protect the laceration. You'll also get a step-by-step demonstration of how to apply a traction splint to a patient with a broken femur, and I'll even show you how to build your own traction splint with nothing more than a ski pole, a few carabiners and some nylon webbing and 550 cord (or whatever else you happen to have in your backpack).

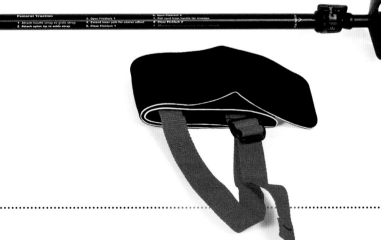

SEVERE BLEEDING

Severe, life-threatening bleeding is something beyond what most people have seen. Those of us with young children know that in their minds, a scraped knee or pinprick constitutes serious bleeding. But a major arterial bleed is usually characterized by spurting or spraying blood, blood that has a "pulse" (in other words, when the heart beats, blood gushes or sprays out) and blood that is bright red from being highly oxygenated. My first encounter with a serious arterial bleed was a patient with a laceration to the brachial artery, which resulted in a column of blood the thickness of pencil lead spraying 3 feet and splashing back off the wall it hit. While less-serious bleeding should still be cared for, a serious arterial bleed, such as an injury from a gunshot or a stab wound, can end a patient's life in minutes. Because of this, it's going to take precedence over any other item on our assessment checklist discussed in Chapter 1.

Field Treatment

In order to stop serious arterial bleeding, you'll need to immediately provide direct, significant pressure to the injury. Direct pressure can be applied with nothing more than a gloved hand, but a better solution, and something that will promote clotting, would be sterile surgical gauze, a hemostatic dressing or a compression bandage. We'll hit each of those one at a time.

Sterile Gauze or Surgical Sponge

Let's start with nothing more complex than a stack of sterile gauze, or surgical sponges. In the event of serious bleeding, immediate, direct pressure is critical, even if another individual is preparing a more advanced intervention, such as a tourniquet. Once pressure has been applied, do not remove the gauze or sponge to check the injury, and if the gauze or sponge becomes soaked in blood, simply layer more gauze or another sponge on top and continue the direct pressure.

Hemostatic Dressing

Serious bleeding can also be controlled by using a hemostatic dressing, such as a QuikClot or Celox sponge. While not cheap, hemostatic sponges are similar in thickness to surgical sponges, but they are impregnated with a compound that absorbs the fluid in blood, leading to more rapid clotting than with a surgical sponge or gauze alone. Hemostatic dressings work through a physical, rather than chemical, reaction by rapidly absorbing the water molecules contained in blood, leading to the clotting action. If you have immediate access to a hemostatic dressing, it should be placed first, directly on top of (or packed into) the wound, with direct pressure applied for two to three minutes, which allows the clotting action to take effect. After the bleeding has been controlled, a compression bandage can be placed next, holding the hemostatic dressing in place and applying additional pressure. Hemostatic solutions from QuikClot and Celox include sponges, z-folded gauze (which is valuable if a deep penetrating wound must be packed tightly to control the bleeding) and granules that can be poured directly into the wound. Celox has even developed a solution called the Celox-A applicator, which is a pre-packed, large-bore syringe containing 6 grams of Celox granules. This solution allows the hemostatic granules to be injected deep into a penetrating injury, allowing the granules to reach the source of the bleeding.

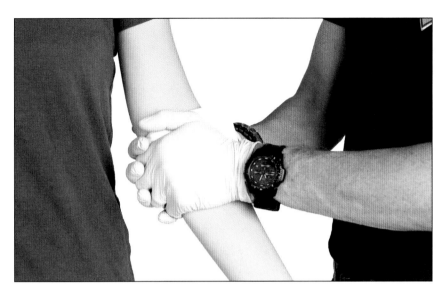

■ Surgical Gauze or Sponge

In the event of serious bleeding, immediate, direct pressure is critical, even if another individual is preparing a more advanced intervention, such as a tourniquet. After pressure has been applied, do not remove the gauze or sponge to check the injury, and if the gauze or sponge becomes soaked in blood, simply layer more gauze or another sponge on top and continue the direct pressure.

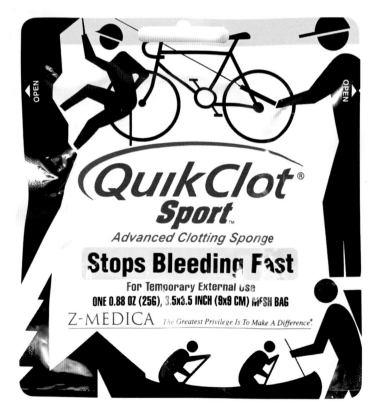

■ QuikClot Sponge

QuikClot and other hemostatic sponges are impregnated with a compound that absorbs the fluid in blood, leading to more rapid clotting than with a surgical sponge or gauze alone. Hemostatic sponges work through a physical, rather than chemical, reaction by rapidly absorbing the water molecules contained in blood, leading to the clotting action. If you have immediate access to a hemostatic dressing, it should be placed first, directly on top of (or packed into) the wound, with direct pressure applied for two to three minutes, which allows the clotting action to take effect.

Compression Bandages

While there are a number of products that I recommend you include in your own emergency first-aid kit (much more on this topic in Chapter 4), a pressure bandage is at the top of my list. I've got two favorites: the emergency bandage (or Israeli bandage as it's also known) and the "H" bandage.

The Emergency Bandage

The emergency bandage is simple in design. Through the use of an elasticized wrapping and a plastic pressure plate, the emergency bandage is able to apply many times the pressure applied by traditional gauze wrapping alone. To use the emergency bandage, remove it from its outer and inner packaging and place the thick sterile pad directly over the injury. Pulling tightly to stretch the elastic, you'll wrap it around the limb once and then loop it through the pressure plate. You'll then reverse direction, again pulling tightly to maximize the pressure, and you'll continue to wrap the limb, overlapping above, below and on each side of the injury.

When applied correctly, the elasticized wrapping will put a great deal of pressure on the injury, which will slow the bleeding or stop it altogether. The trick with all compression bandages is to concentrate on pulling the wrapping good and tight with each revolution. While your patient might complain that you're wrapping it too tightly, the alternative may be that the artery continues to bleed uncontrolled.

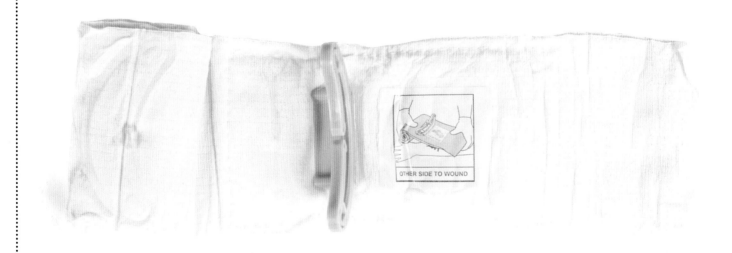

OTHER SIDE TO WOUND

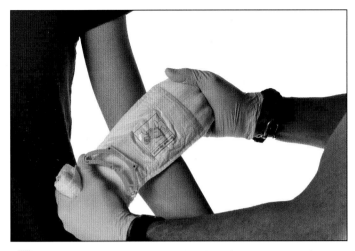

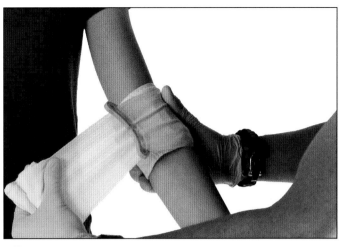

Step 1: Remove the emergency bandage from its outer and inner packaging and open it up to place the thick sterile pad directly over the injury.

Step 2: Pull tightly to stretch the elastic and wrap it around the limb once. Then loop the elastic wrap through the pressure plate.

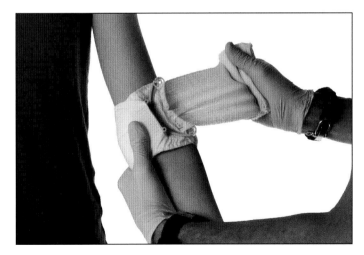

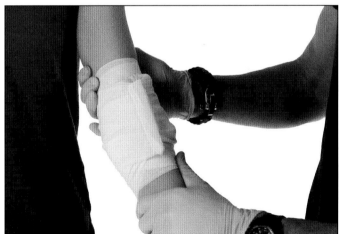

Step 3: Reverse direction, pulling tightly to maximize the pressure. Continue to wrap the limb, overlapping above, below and on each side of the injury.

Step 4: Secure the bandage in place with the plastic retaining lock.

The "H" Bandage

I have to say that the "H" bandage (named after the "H"-shaped pressure plate on its face) just edges out the emergency bandage as my favorite compression dressing. Like the emergency bandage, the "H" bandage has a plastic pressure plate which is placed directly over the injury. But the "H" bandage also allows multiple passes of the elasticized bandage to be looped through and around the pressure plate, adding additional pressure with each pass. The "H" bandage adds the convenience of Velcro on the first 12 inches, which holds the bandage temporarily in place while you're getting it positioned, and another at the tail end, which holds the wrapped bandage in place while you're preparing to secure it with the plastic retaining lock. I also appreciate the fact that the "H" bandage comes in a single wrapper, which is easily torn open along the pre-cut notch, allowing for rapid deployment. I have yet to open an emergency bandage from its outer and inner wrapper without using my trauma shears, which can cost precious seconds. The "H" bandage is applied using the procedure as shown on the opposite page.

If direct pressure or compression bandages aren't stopping the bleeding or if the bleeding is so severe that you need to immediately get more aggressive (for example, in the case of an amputated limb or if the laceration is too long to be able to apply the proper pressure), you'll need to step up to a tourniquet, explained next.

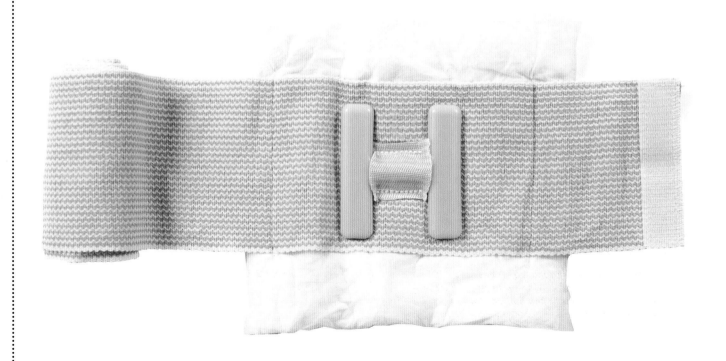

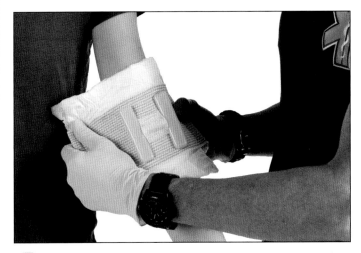

Step 1: Remove the "H" bandage from its outer packaging and open it up to place the thick, sterile pad directly over the injury.

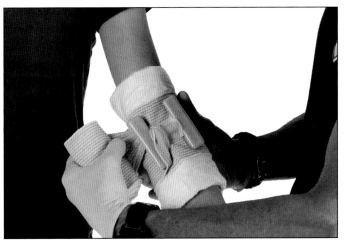

Step 2: Pull tightly to stretch the elastic and wrap it around the limb once (a velcro tab on the back of the bandage will hold it in place while you position it). Loop the elastic wrap around one side of the "H," then pull tightly and reverse direction.

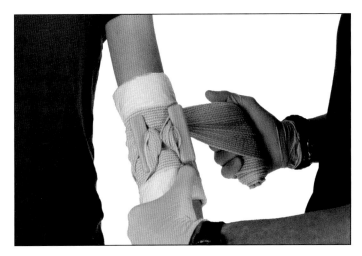

Step 3: Loop the bandage around the other side of the "H." Reverse direction again and continue wrapping. Loops may continue to be added to the "H" to add additional pressure. After completing loops around the "H," continue to wrap the limb, overlapping above, below and on each side of the injury.

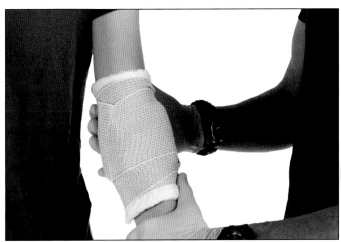

Step 4: Secure the bandage in place with the plastic retaining lock.

Tourniquets

Anyone who attended an advanced first-aid course in the '80s or '90s was most likely instructed that tourniquets were not even a method of last resort. They were a method that should *never* be resorted to because they risked permanently damaging major blood vessels and could result in the loss of a limb.

The belief was that since other options could usually stem the flow of blood from even serious lacerations, if tourniquets were taught as an option, they'd be used inappropriately. But 10 years of war in Iraq and Afghanistan taught a different story. It not only became apparent that the use of a tourniquet could save the life of a patient when no other option was working but also demonstrated that even moderately trained individuals were smart enough to only apply a tourniquet when it was medically necessary.

A 2008 study reviewed tourniquet use in Iraq in 2006, where 232 patients had 428 tourniquets applied on 309 injured limbs. Researchers concluded that tourniquets

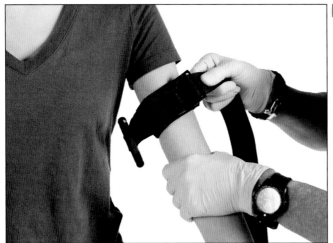

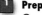 **Prepare and Position the Tourniquet**

Open the strap wide enough to fit the limb through it or disconnect the slip-gate buckle from the strap by twisting it free from the U-shaped clip, wrap it around the limb and reconnect the slip-gate to the strap.

Place the tourniquet between the injury and the heart (not on a joint), and pull the strap tight.

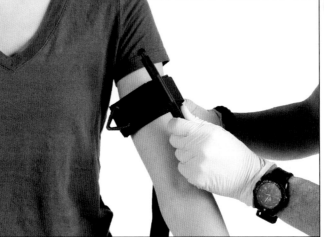

 Twist Until Bleeding Stops

Twist the aluminum windlass until the bleeding stops. Your patient may complain that the tourniquet is hurting him or her, but if the artery is continuing to bleed, it isn't tight enough.

were medically necessary in 97 percent of the cases, or in all but 12 of the 428 applied tourniquets. That same study addressed the concern that tourniquet use would result in the loss of limbs or that extended use of a tourniquet would damage nerves or cause blood clots, leading to the patient's death. The study found that the average tourniquet time was 1.3 hours, yet the researchers concluded that "no amputations resulted solely from tourniquet use." In one case, a tourniquet remained applied for 14 hours, yet that patient survived.

Modern tourniquets, such as the SOF Tactical Tourniquet (Wide) (SOFTT-W), the Combat Application Tourniquet (CAT) and the Ratcheting Medical Tourniquet (RMT), are battlefield-proven and are each designed to be quickly deployed either by a rescuer or to be self-applied. The example below demonstrates how to properly apply the SOFTT-W on an upper extremity.

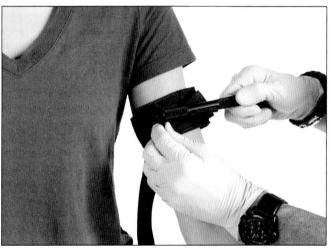

Lock the Windlass
Lock the windlass in place using the triangular locking buckle.

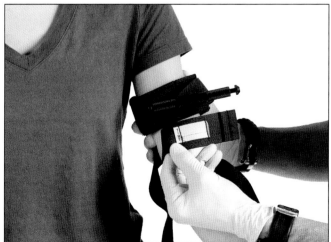

Record Time
Note the time that you placed the tourniquet on the white tag, which will be valuable information for emergency room staff. Under no circumstances should you loosen or remove the tourniquet!

Tourniquet Review

While a variety of commercial tourniquets are available, the four most popular include the SOFTT, the SOFTT-W, the CAT and the RMT. The overview below provides a bit more detail about how they work, as well as their pros and cons. I've also scored them from 1 to 5 (5 being the highest) on their ability to deploy easily and quickly, on their ability to be deployed one-handed (something that you'll find important if you're the one who has the severe arterial bleed and no one is around to help you), and on their ease of disconnecting the strap from the buckle, which is helpful when placing the tourniquet around a lower extremity and is required when the extremity is pinned under an immovable object.

▶ Combat Application Tourniquet

Now in its 7th generation, the CAT has a proven track record that's tough to match (and most likely won't be matched until the U.S. finds itself in another armed conflict). The CAT is applied by loosening the Velcro strap (or removing the strap from the friction buckle), placing it in position and pre-tightening it by pulling the strap tight and reapplying the Velcro. To tighten, the windless is turned in either direction until the bleeding stops. To lock the windlass in place, drop it into the C-shaped cradle (the tension of the windlass will lock it in place). Cover the locking cradle with the white Velcro strip, which also doubles as a place to record the time of application. Deploying the CAT one-handed on a model prior to the 7th generation is troublesome unless it is preconfigured into one-handed mode, which involves routing the Velcro strap through just one of the buckle's two gates. That allows the operator to pre-tighten the CAT by pulling the strap straight out from the body before locking the Velcro strap back onto itself. The 7th generation solves that problem by using a buckle with a single, rather than a double, gate. Some users dislike the Velcro strap, which can occasionally lock onto itself at precisely the wrong moment (such as when trying to remove the strap from the friction buckle), and the windlass is plastic, which has been known to break.

5 Speed of Application

4 Ease of Deploying One-Handed

4 Ease of Disconnecting Strap From Buckle

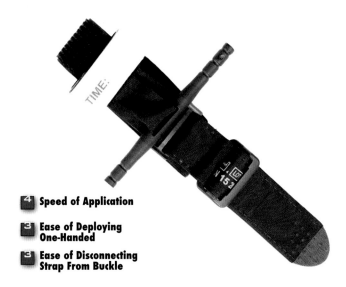

4 Speed of Application

3 Ease of Deploying One-Handed

3 Ease of Disconnecting Strap From Buckle

◀ SOF Tactical Tourniquet

The SOFTT operates much like the CAT, but instead of using a Velcro strap to hold it in place as it's being pre-tightened, the SOFTT uses a toothed buckle and a tension thumbscrew that must be loosened to pre-tighten the strap and then screwed down to lock the strap in place (and to keep the strap from slipping when the windlass is turned). Like the CAT, the SOFTT is tightened by turning the windlass until the bleeding stops. To lock the windlass in place, one or both of the triangular buckles are locked over the end of the windlass. At the tag end of the strap is a white label, which is used to record the time of application. Unlike the CAT, there is no need to configure the SOFTT any differently for one-handed versus two-handed use since the strap will slip easily through the toothed buckle when self-applying on an upper extremity (assuming that the tension thumbscrew isn't locked down tight). The SOFTT also allows the strap to be completely freed from the toothed buckle by pressing the tension thumbscrew, which raises the teeth from the buckle, allowing the strap to be quickly pulled free.

▶ SOF Tactical Tourniquet (Wide)

The SOFTT-W is an improvement on the already trusted SOFTT, with a strap that's 1.5 inches wide (compared to 1 inch on the SOFTT). The SOFTT-W also does away with the tension thumbscrew and replaces it with a slip-gate buckle. The SOFTT-W is applied by loosening the strap (if necessary) and placing it in position. Where the SOFTT-W really shines is in its simple ability to disconnect the slip-gate buckle from the strap by twisting it free from the U-shaped clip. This is a major benefit when sliding the tourniquet up an arm or leg is impractical or impossible. After placing the tourniquet in position, the slip-gate buckle is clipped back in place and the tag end of the strap is tightened. Like the CAT and SOFTT, the SOFTT-W is tightened by turning the windlass until the bleeding stops. The SOFTT-W has just a single triangular-shaped lock rather than the two on the SOFTT, but one is plenty. The time of application may also be recorded on the white tag on the end of the strap.

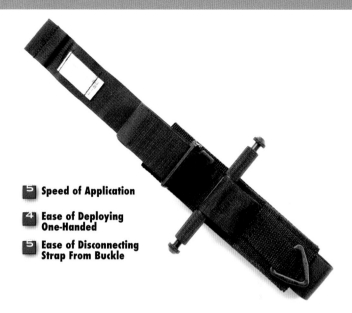

5 Speed of Application

4 Ease of Deploying One-Handed

5 Ease of Disconnecting Strap From Buckle

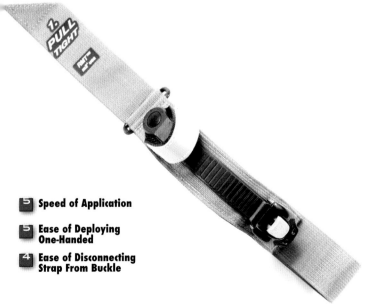

5 Speed of Application

5 Ease of Deploying One-Handed

4 Ease of Disconnecting Strap From Buckle

◀ Ratcheting Medical Tourniquet

The RMT is the most innovative tourniquet to hit the market in years and is gaining a huge following in law enforcement, EMS and the military. The application of the RMT will be immediately apparent to anyone who has slipped on a pair of roller blades or ski boots that are tightened with ratcheting straps. After positioning the tourniquet, it can be pre-tightened by grasping the "bite strap" with an index finger and pulling the tag end tight. If you're wondering why the bite strap is so named, it's because it aids in self-application on an upper extremity when it's necessary to apply the tourniquet one-handed. The operator simply slides the RMT into place, bites the "bite strap" and pre-tightens the strap by pulling it tight. To tighten the RMT, the operator simply lifts up on the black ratchet until the bleeding stops (you get to hear that satisfying "click" just like you'd expect). Since the ratchet (by design) is always locked in place, nothing further must be done. To release, lift up on the coyote colored tab inside of the ratchet. The RMT is available with straps 1.5 or 2 inches wide, with other models designed specifically for pediatric and even K9 use.

MAINTENANCE OF A LACERATION

As mentioned in the introduction, one difference that exists between professional EMS rescuers and nonprofessionals is that the professionals rarely have to worry about maintaining a patient's condition for more than half an hour (and it's frequently less time than that, with metro area hospitals usually no more than 10 to 15 minutes away). Nonprofessionals, on the other hand, especially when they find themselves miles from civilization at the family cabin or on a camping, hunting or canoe trip, might find it necessary to not only stop severe bleeding if a companion becomes injured but also maintain the stability and health of the laceration until help arrives. When it comes to severe lacerations, I'm going to recommend just four additional steps if you find yourself more than eight hours from rescue. Less time than that, and the steps you've already taken should suffice. More time than that, and you risk serious infection unless the injury is properly cleaned and protected. Let's start with cleansing of the laceration, which accounts for Step 1 and Step 2.

1. Cleaning the Wound Hydraulically

One of the simplest and least-invasive methods of cleansing a wound is to clean it hydraulically, which is a fancy way of saying you should clean it by squirting sterile water into the wound. The first bit of preparation needs to occur before you leave home, and that's to include a large-volume syringe with a screw-on plastic tip and a foil package of povidone-iodine (used to create the sterile solution as explained on the right) in your emergency first-aid kit. Lacking a syringe, I suggest two field-expedient options on the opposite page using

a water bottle or a plastic bag. If you haven't packed povidone-iodine, you'll need to sterilize a gallon of water by boiling it for one to three minutes. Allow the water to cool enough so that it won't burn the patient and then spray the sterilized water or the povidone-iodine mixture into the laceration, dislodging and removing any foreign contaminants.

2. Scrub the Wound Clean

After that procedure is complete, a more aggressive cleansing can occur by using a povidone-iodine mixture, water that you've sterilized or an over-the-counter wound cleaner. Spray your solution onto sterile gauze and then carefully scrub the wound to remove any additional contaminants. This will hurt, so warn your patient about what you're going to do and then complete the procedure quickly.

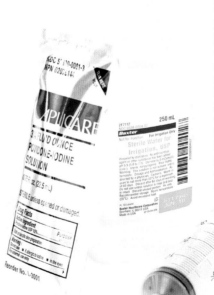

Povidone-Iodine Mixture
While water sterilized by boiling will work for hydraulic cleansing of a wound, if you want to add a couple items to your medium or large first-aid kit, you can include a 250-ml bottle of sterile water and a 0.75-ounce foil package of povidone-iodine (10%). Mix the povidone-iodine with the sterile water and you've got the same sterile mixture used in operating rooms around the world. Besides being more sterile, it means you also get to skip lighting a fire.

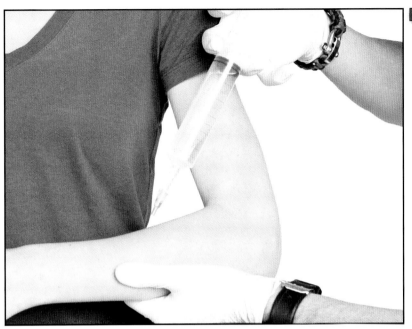

Flush the Wound

While wearing a pair of nitrile gloves, squirt the sterilized water or povidone-iodine mixture into the laceration, dislodging and removing any foreign contaminants. This step may need to be performed a number of times to remove all contaminants.

Field-Expedient Syringe

Lacking a large-volume syringe, a field-expedient version can be created by taking a standard water bottle and melting a hole in the cap with a safety pin heated with a match or lighter. Fill the bottle with your sterile solution, then squeeze the bottle to forcefully spray it into the laceration. Don't have a water bottle or a safety pin? An even more rudimentary solution is to poke a pinhole into any plastic bag. Fill the bag with your sterile solution, then squeeze the bag like a pastry chef would to forcefully spray the solution into the laceration to dislodge any contaminants.

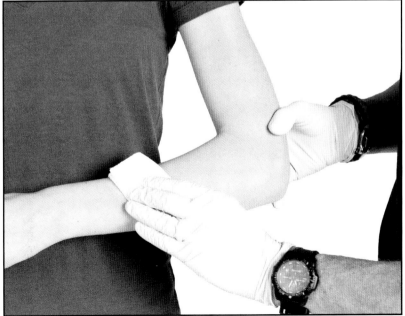

Scrub the Wound

Spray your povidone-iodine mixture, your sterile water or an over-the-counter wound cleaner onto sterile gauze and then carefully scrub the wound to remove any remaining contaminants.

3. Wound Closing

Wound closing should only be considered if your patient is more than eight hours from rescue. While invasive wound closure devices are available over the counter (or over the internet) without a prescription, I'm going to recommend that you leave suture kits and skin staple guns to the professionals. A great alternative to traditional sutures are adhesive sutures, such as the 3M Steri-Strips shown here. Adhesive sutures are thin strips of sterile tape which are placed perpendicular across a laceration, holding it closed.

This solution is more practical for straight, cleanly cut lacerations (such as what might occur from a knife or ax wound) but are less practical for large open wounds (such as what might occur from a gunshot wound or a crush injury). For those injuries, I'd recommend skipping the closing step and moving on to the protecting step.

4. Protecting the Wound

The last step that should be accomplished when dealing with a significant laceration is to protect the wound by covering it with a sterile dressing. While a large piece of sterile gauze can be taped in place, that's likely to eventually work its way loose, allowing contaminants to enter the laceration. A better solution is to use a gel bandage, such as the 3M Tegaderm Film shown here, which adheres to the skin all around the laceration, sealing out contaminants without bonding too tightly to the laceration itself. A gel bandage also promotes healing and is clear, which allows the laceration to be inspected for infection without removing the bandage.

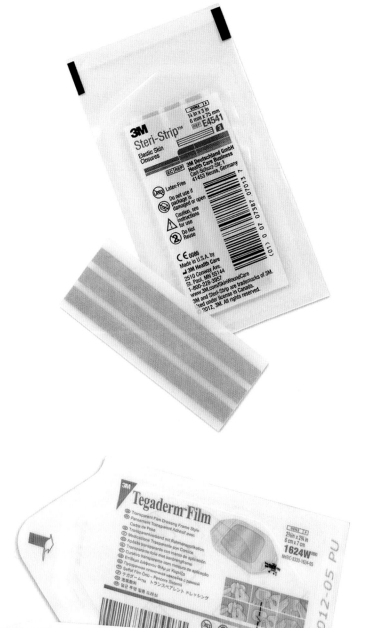

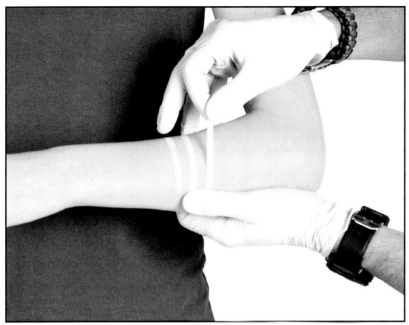

 Close the Wound
Carefully place the sutures perpendicular across the laceration, ensuring that the edges of the laceration have been carefully pulled together. Place additional sutures approximately every half-inch until the entire laceration has been closed.

If you'd like to dramatically increase the adhesiveness of sutures, tape and even moleskin, see Chapter 4 for an explanation of why you should consider adding **Benzoin Swabs** to your personal emergency first-aid kit.

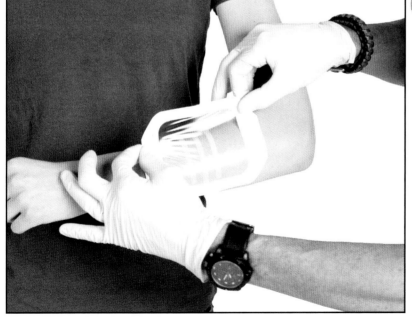

 Protect the Wound
Place a large gel bandage directly over the sutured laceration. A gel bandage will allow you to observe the injury for continued bleeding or signs of infection, and it will promote healing.

PENETRATING CHEST INJURIES

When it comes to the ABCs of airway, breathing and circulation, it's easy to recognize that a blocked airway, a lack of breathing, a stopped heart or severe bleeding will compromise those ABCs and that death can result unless the compromise is quickly corrected. What may not be as obvious but can be equally as deadly are injuries to

[hi-**pok**-see-uh]
A deficiency in the amount of oxygen reaching the tissues of the body.

the chest, including penetrating injuries. A penetrating injury to the chest is an extremely serious injury that will severely compromise your patient's ability to achieve a proper volume of breathing, ultimately leading to a lack of oxygenated blood to the body (most importantly, the brain), or what EMS would call "**hypoxia**."

Open Pneumothorax

A penetrating injury to the front or back of the torso that has penetrated at least to the pleural space (the layer between the lungs and the chest wall) is referred to as an open pneumothorax. To understand what a pneumothorax is and why it's so dangerous, you have to first understand a bit about the mechanics of breathing. Ask the average person why the chest rises on inspiration (when a person breathes in), and he or she would most likely say that it expands because the lungs fill with air, much the same as how a balloon inflates when air is blown into it. But that's actually incorrect, and the opposite is true. The chest doesn't rise because

the lungs fill with air; the lungs fill with air because the chest rises. Let me explain that a bit further. The chest wall (and the lungs along with it) expands due to the diaphragm and the intercostal muscles (the muscles between the ribs) both contracting. According to Boyle's Law, the expanded volume results in decreased pressure inside of the lungs. Air then rushes into the airway to equalize the lower pressure inside the lungs with the higher pressure outside the lungs. On expiration (when the person breathes out), the diaphragm and intercostal muscles relax, and the elastic recoil of the chest increases pressure in the lungs, causing the air to rush out of the airway. In order for the lungs to expand as the chest wall expands, a vacuum must be maintained in the pleural space (there is actually no connecting tissue between the chest wall and the lungs, only a small amount of fluid to reduce friction). When the vacuum in this space is lost due to a penetrating injury, the lung will separate from the chest wall during inspiration, and Boyle's Law once again takes effect as air rushes into the pleural space to equalize the pressure. A pneumothorax results. Even a small amount of air in the pleural space will dramatically increase respiratory effort, which in turn can lead to hypoxia. Larger volumes of air in this space can lead to what's referred to as a "tension pneumothorax," or the pleural space completely filling with air. This causes the lung to collapse and pressure on the heart to increase dramatically, which can reduce

[numo-**thor**-ax]
A condition where air has entered the pleural space and the vacuum in this space is lost.

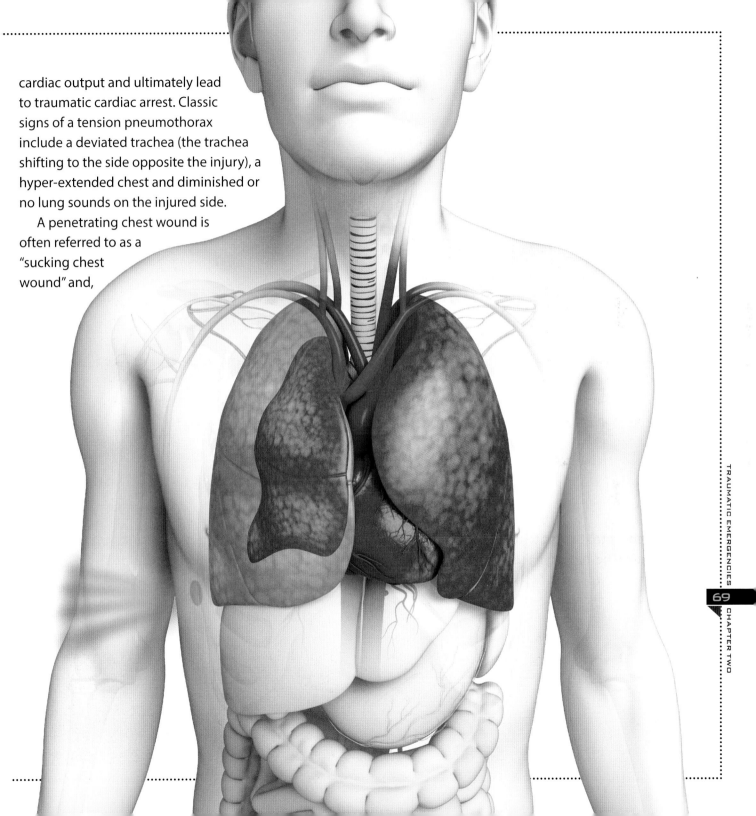

cardiac output and ultimately lead to traumatic cardiac arrest. Classic signs of a tension pneumothorax include a deviated trachea (the trachea shifting to the side opposite the injury), a hyper-extended chest and diminished or no lung sounds on the injured side.

A penetrating chest wound is often referred to as a "sucking chest wound" and, to be honest, it's a great descriptive term for how to identify this type of injury. As the nickname implies, this type of injury can be identified not just by the apparent penetration to the upper torso but also by the "sucking" sound as air enters and leaves the wound.

Field Treatment

While there is no nonprofessional treatment in the field that can manually extract air from the pleural space, there *is* a field-expedient treatment that can limit the amount of additional air that leaks into this space as the patient breathes in and allow air to escape as the patient breathes out.

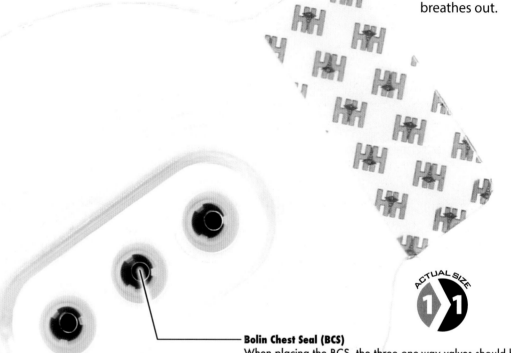

Bolin Chest Seal (BCS)
When placing the BCS, the three one-way valves should be positioned directly over the penetration to the upper torso. The seal will re-establish the vacuum in the pleural space, and the valves will allow air to leak out of the space when the patient breathes out and will prevent additional air from entering the space when the patient breathes in. If signs and symptoms of a pneumothorax develop, the seal can be "burped" by lifting up the tab and allowing air to vent out of the space before reapplying the seal.

OCCLUSIVE

[ah-**clue**-siv]
A dressing that blocks air from passing through it.

This is done by creating a one-way valve over the injury by taping a piece of plastic (such as a sandwich bag) over the injury on three sides. The open side will allow air to leak out of the pleural space when the patient breathes out but will limit or eliminate additional air entering the space when the patient breathes in. It can also re-establish the necessary vacuum. But for a far superior option, I recommend that for a large first-aid kit (the type you'd bring along when you're more than a day from EMS coverage, as you'd be on a multi-day hiking, camping or canoeing trip), you include a commercial chest seal, designed specifically to deal with penetrating chest wounds. Chest seals are round or oval, with adhesive on one side and a one-way valve on the other side (although some chest seals lack the valve and are **occlusive** — more on that topic in the next section). When applying a chest seal, the valve(s) should be placed directly over the penetrating injury. In the case of a gunshot wound, you may have to place two seals: one on the entry wound and one on the exit wound. For the full field treatment of a penetrating wound to the chest, see the emergency care procedures explained on the right.

SUCKING CHEST WOUND

EMERGENCY CARE

Here's what you should do if you find yourself with a patient who has sustained a sucking chest wound:

- Upon identifying the sucking chest wound, immediately cover it with a gloved hand. Covering it with the back of your hand leaves your fingers free to prepare a chest seal.
- If the penetrating injury is due to a gunshot wound, immediately check the opposite side of the patient for an exit wound.
- Use a clean towel or sterile gauze to wipe the immediate area clean of blood, sweat or other fluids that might interfere with a tight seal.
- If using a commercial seal, remove the backing and prepare to place the seal. If the seal has a valve, the valve should be placed directly over the penetrating injury. If an exit wound exists, place a second seal over that injury. Apply the seal at the moment of full expiration.
- If creating a field-expedient seal, place an occlusive covering (such as a sandwich bag or other plastic bag) over the injury and tape it on three sides. The open side allows the trapped air to "burp" out while eliminating the introduction of additional air into the pleural space.
- Monitor the patient for signs and symptoms of a tension pneumothorax, and "burp" the seal if they appear.

A CHEST SEAL PRIMER
WHAT'S BETTER: A VENTED OR NON-VENTED CHEST SEAL?

Like many product innovations designed to deal with severe trauma, chest seals were born out of battlefield necessity, with penetrating chest trauma with lung perforation accounting for 5 to 6 percent of battlefield injuries. As explained earlier, a penetrating chest wound creates significant risks to the patient by causing the required vacuum within the pleural space to be lost as air enters the space, creating what's referred to as an "open pneumothorax." On the battlefield, the accepted treatment was to tape an occlusive (air-tight) dressing over the injury on three sides, effectively creating a one-way valve, allowing air to escape from the pleural space while reintroducing a vacuum (negative pressure). However, with no formal study to back up this method of treatment, the U.S. Military Committee on Tactical Combat Casualty Care (TCCC) subsequently recommended that these battlefield injuries be treated by covering them in a completely occlusive (non-vented) chest seal while closely monitoring patients for signs of a tension pneumothorax. If signs and symptoms became apparent, untrained personnel were taught to "burp" the chest seal, allowing trapped air to escape, while trained medics could treat the condition by inserting a chest decompression needle and venting off the trapped air.

Evidence for vented versus non-vented chest seals remained anecdotal until a 2013 study in San Antonio, where vented and non-vented seals were tested to compare their ability to reduce respiratory effort and prevent or reduce the chances of a tension pneumothorax from developing. Using sedated Yorkshire pigs (which approximate human anatomy), researchers created an 11.5-mm penetration through the chest wall, simulating a gunshot wound or other penetrating injury. Air was allowed to flow freely through the penetration into the pleural space, resulting in intrapleural pressure moving from negative to at or near zero.

During this time, the respiratory rate and tidal volume (the amount of air entering the lungs) dropped, as did the saturated oxygen in the blood. Cardiac output remained relatively stable. After five minutes, a chest seal was applied. The results of the tests concluded that vented and non-vented chest seals provided an immediate reduction in respiratory effort, and both seals returned most vitals to near-baseline levels when measured five minutes after they were applied. In other words, both chest seals worked equally as well.

Where the seals diverged however, was when the researchers introduced additional air into the pleural space through a syringe and catheter, which was used to simulate what would occur if the lung wall itself were also penetrated, allowing air to continue to leak into the pleural space internally (even though the external penetration was blocked by a chest seal). When using non-vented chest seals, intrapleural pressure continued to increase, tidal volume and cardiac output decreased, and saturated oxygen levels fell below 60 percent (a hypoxic level at which the brain can no longer function). Respiratory effort in all subjects became more strenuous, and a tension pneumothorax developed in all subjects (and respiratory arrest occurred in some of the subjects) when the intrapleural pressure reached +10 mm Hg (millimeters of mercury).

However, when using vented seals, vital signs, including respiratory rate, tidal volume, saturated oxygen and cardiac output, remained stable, even when the maximum amount of air (a volume equal to the amount of total lung capacity of the subject) was injected into the pleural space.

The study concluded, and the U.S. Military's TCCC agreed, that vented chest seals provided a superior ability to reduce the chances of a tension pneumothorax in patients with penetrating chest injuries. However, vented chest seals should not be viewed as a panacea, and even patients treated with a vented chest seal must still be monitored for signs and symptoms of a tension pneumothorax.

As the study also indicated, non-vented chest seals will still provide a reduction in respiratory effort; however, if signs or symptoms of a tension pneumothorax develop, the seal will need to be "burped," as will a vented chest seal if the valve or valves have become occluded with blood.

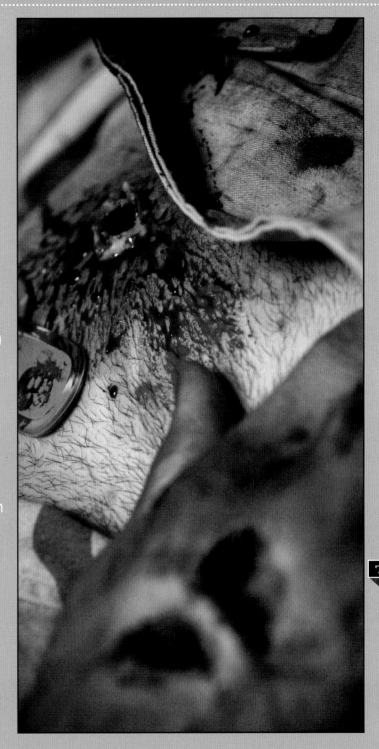

Chest Seal Options

While vented and non-vented chest seals are commercially available, as explained in the preceding section, vented chest seals are considered superior for their ability to reduce or prevent a tension pneumothorax in patients with penetrating chest injuries. However, non-vented chest seals are still appropriate for these types of injuries if EMS is no more than five minutes away or when no vented chest seal is available. I've provided an overview of each of the chest

➡ H&H Bolin Chest Seal (BCS)

I like just about anything produced by H&H, and the Bolin Chest Seal (BCS) is no exception. It's a standard addition in Chinook Trauma kits for good reason. The vented BCS avoids clogging by tripling-down on one-way valves, which will allow air to continue to vent even if one or two valves becomes clogged with blood. The BCS is made from polyurethane and is incredibly flexible, allowing the seal to be molded over the contours of the chest with no wrinkles or gaps. The BCS uses a jelly-based adhesive that significantly outperformed the Asherman Chest Seal (ACS) in adhesive qualities on blood-soiled skin during a test conducted by the Naval Medical Research Center. This thick adhesive helps the BCS to stick and remain stuck to a patient even in the most extreme environments and situations — all while still allowing the seal to be "burped" if all three valves become occluded and the patient begins to show signs of a tension pneumothorax. If the BCS has any benefit over the SAM Chest Seal (opposite page), it's that its thinner valves allow thinner packaging, which means it can be rolled and squeezed into a typical trauma kit.

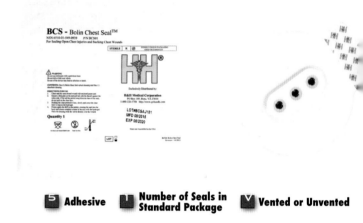

5 **Adhesive**   2 **Number of Seals in Standard Package**   V **Vented or Unvented**

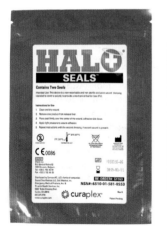

 Adhesive   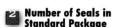 **Number of Seals in Standard Package**   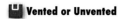 **Vented or Unvented**

◀ HALO Chest Seal

HALO unvented chest seals have been a standard of the U.S. military for a number of years due to their simple design and adhesive qualities. Like the BCS and SAM, the HALO uses a gel-based adhesive, although it is noticeably thinner than the adhesive layers on the BCS and SAM. As discussed in the chest seal primer, the U.S. Military Committee on Tactical Combat Casualty Care (TCCC) had previously recommended that the occlusive properties of the HALO and other unvented chest seals were preferable to vented seals, but that recommendation has been reversed based upon the 2013 San Antonio study. That said, the occlusive HALO will provide an immediate reduction in respiratory effort for a patient with a sucking chest wound, and the HALO is the only chest seal which contains two seals per package, which will be incredibly valuable if dealing with an entry *and* an exit wound. When using the HALO, if signs of a tension pneumothorax develop, it can be easily "burped" and resealed.

seals below, and I've also scored them from 1 to 5 on their adhesive ability (that is, how well the seal is able to adhere to skin that may be bloody or sweaty). If the seal is unvented, I've indicated that with a "U." Vented seals are indicated with a "V." Finally, each chest seal below will receive a "1" if the package contains one seal or a "2" if the package contains two seals. Having two seals will be ultra important in the case of a gunshot injury with an entrance *and* an exit wound.

▶ SAM Chest Seal (With Valve)

SAM Medical has two versions of chest seals available: one vented and one unvented. The vented seal contains a domed vent with a cap. When the cap is in place, the seal is occlusive (in other words, it acts as an unvented seal), and when the cap is removed, the one-way valve is activated, allowing air trapped within the pleural space to escape while preventing more air from entering. The dome design of the vent has two benefits. First, the valve vents out to the side of the dome through four ports rather than venting through the center, so it won't be blocked by a blanket or other covering. Second, the domed interior helps to avoid blockage by blood and fluids. Like the BCS, the SAM seal is made from thick polyurethane and has a "rubberized" feel, which allows it to fit the contours of the chest, and the gel-based adhesive is very thick and extremely tacky. It's the best adhesive among the bunch, allowing it to stick through blood, sweat, hair, dirt or sand. It can also be "burped" and resealed multiple times. If there is any downside at all, it's that the domed valve makes the packaging thicker, making it more difficult to fit in a prepackaged trauma kit. Rescuers must be aware that when the cap is in place, no venting of the pleural space will occur.

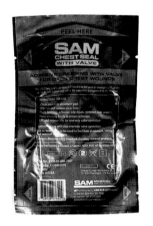
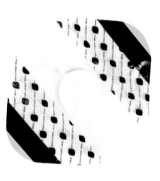

5 Adhesive   **1** Number of Seals in Standard Package   **V** Vented or Unvented

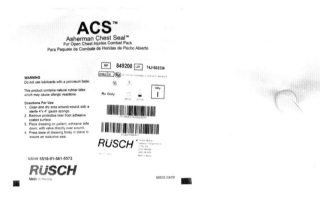

◀ Asherman Chest Seal (ACS)

Unlike the BCS or SAM, the Asherman Chest Seal (ACS) uses a more rudimentary flutter valve that acts similar to the mouth of a balloon. While extremely simple in design, this style of valve is more susceptible to clogging from blood than the triple-valve design of the BCS or the domed design of the SAM. At 5.5 inches in diameter, the ACS is also the smallest seal of the bunch. There is one upside though: It's the least expensive among the four seals at about $12 retail.

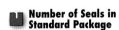
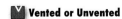

3 Adhesive   **1** Number of Seals in Standard Package   **V** Vented or Unvented

MAJOR BURNS

A major burn is one of the most serious injuries that can occur, even when under the umbrella of EMS coverage. If you encounter a patient with a serious burn when more than a few minutes away from emergency care, you'll need to provide immediate treatment to minimize the long-term risk to the patient. Three criteria are important to evaluate on a burn patient: the depth, extent and location of the burn.

Depth

We've all heard burns referred to as "Second Degree" or "Third Degree" on dozens of TV dramas, but what exactly do those terms mean, and how much more serious is a third-degree burn than a second-degree burn? As shown on the illustration, burns are categorized as first, second or third degree based upon which layer of skin the burn has destroyed. Using more modern terminology, these burns are referred to as "superficial," "partial-thickness" or "full-thickness" burns. Let's look at each of these burn depths in more detail.

First-Degree Burns

Superficial (or first-degree) burns affect just the upper layer of the skin known as the "epidermis." Examples of first-degree burns include sunburn or scald injuries such as you'd receive from momentary contact with boiling water, an open flame or a hot surface. First-degree burns will appear red or pink, and the skin will be dry. Although first-degree burns are superficial in nature, they may be painful since the pain receptors in the underlying dermis layer are still intact. Unless they cover a large area of the body, however, first-degree burns will not typically require emergency medical care unless the patient has a pre-existing condition.

Field Treatment

- Cool the burn with cold water or a cold compress.
- Treat the burn with aloe or another similar product.
- Keep the burn from worsening (e.g. keep the patient from further sun exposure until the burn has healed).

FIRST-DEGREE BURN   SECOND-DEGREE BURN   THIRD-DEGREE BURN

EPIDERMIS

DERMIS

HYPODERMIS

Second-Degree Burns

Also referred to as partial-thickness burns, second-degree burns have not only affected the epidermis but also involve part of the dermis. Since the dermis contains capillaries, damage to this layer will cause plasma to collect between the dermis and epidermis, forming a blister or blisters. These partial-thickness burns will normally cause the skin to appear pink and moist, and they will be extremely painful since the pain receptors in the dermis are directly affected.

Field Treatment

- Immediately remove the condition causing the burn (e.g. burning clothing).
- Cool the burn with continuous cool water.
- Cover the burn in a gel bandage, which will continue to cool the area and promote healing.

Third-Degree Burns

Also referred to as full-thickness burns, third-degree burns have affected all three layers of the skin, including the deepest layer, the hypodermis. Third-degree burns are often caused by prolonged exposure to scalding liquids, extreme heat or open flame, or they may be caused by electrocution. Since most of the nerve endings have been burned away, the full-thickness burn itself may not be painful, but the surrounding tissue will be *extremely* painful. For emergency care for third-degree burns, see the box to the right.

THIRD-DEGREE BURNS

EMERGENCY CARE

- Immediately remove the condition causing the burn (e.g. burning clothing).
- If EMS is more than 24 hours away, you may carefully remove non-adhered clothing and jewelry.
- Assess the burns for depth, extent (using the "rule of nines" as explained on the next page) and location.
- Minor burns (burns covering less than 9 percent of total body surface area) may be treated with wet dressings.
- Major burns (burns covering more than 9 percent of total body surface area) should be covered with a dry sheet. Do <u>not</u> use wet dressings. (We avoid wet dressings when a large surface of the body has received partial- or full-thickness burns because the body's ability to maintain a proper temperature is going to be compromised and we can quickly send our patient into hypothermia if we cool the body too much. Dry dressings can help to avoid that issue.)
- And, finally, closely monitor the patient for signs of shock and hypothermia and to ensure that the airway remains open (particularly for burn injuries near the face).

Extent

The "rule of nines" is a simple way to quickly determine the extent of a burn injury, calculated as a percentage of the total body surface area (TBSA) that has been burned. The body is broken down into blocks of 9 percent, as shown on this page. If more than 9 percent of the body has sustained second- or third-degree burns, use only dry dressings to protect the injuries. Severe burns can compromise the body's ability to regulate temperature, and wet dressings can lead to hypothermia, even in relatively warm conditions.

Location

The location of the burn injury will also affect its seriousness. Burn injuries near the face may have affected the respiratory tract, and circumferential burns around the chest will increase respiratory effort. Circumferential burns around an extremity may cut off circulation beyond the burn. Regardless of burn depth or burn extent, a patient with burns in any of these locations should be immediately evacuated for critical care.

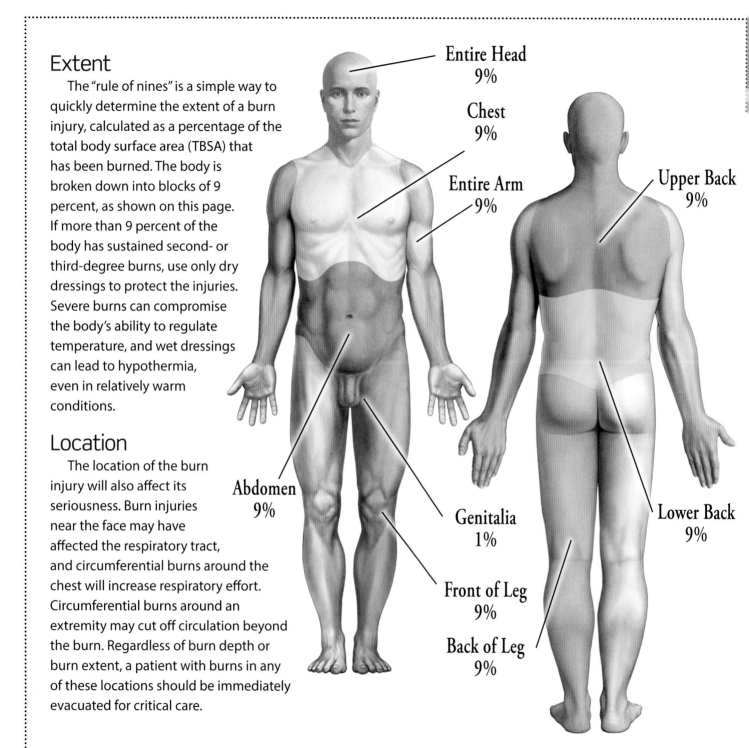

Entire Head
9%

Chest
9%

Entire Arm
9%

Upper Back
9%

Abdomen
9%

Genitalia
1%

Front of Leg
9%

Back of Leg
9%

Lower Back
9%

Commercial Products for Treating Burns

While field-expedient methods of treating partial- or full-thickness burns are available, there are a number of commercially available products, including gel-infused burn dressings (appropriate for second- or third-degree burns covering less than 9 percent of the body) and sterile burn sheets (appropriate for second- or third-degree burns covering more than 9 percent of the body). My favorite products are those from Water-Jel, such as the 4x4 dressing shown below. One or more of these dressings should be a priority item in your emergency first-aid kit.

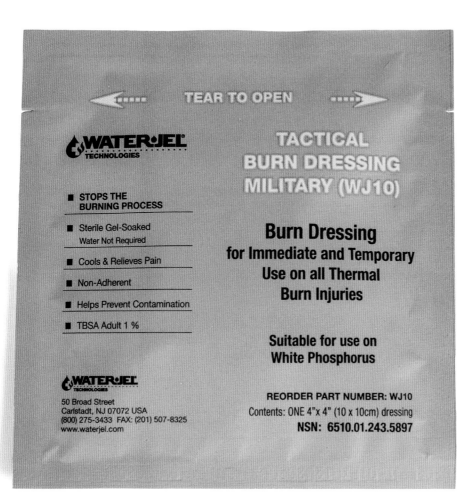

Gel-Infused Burn Dressing
Water-Jel dressings use a gelatinized water mix designed to perform several critical steps for burn management in a single application. Because of their gelatinous nature, they seal the burn from further contamination, and they cool the burn site and relieve pain by absorbing heat. Water-Jel dressings are available in dressings as small as 4x4 inches to as large as 19x11 inches. There are also specialty dressings available for burns to the face or hands and a 5x6-foot dry dressing.

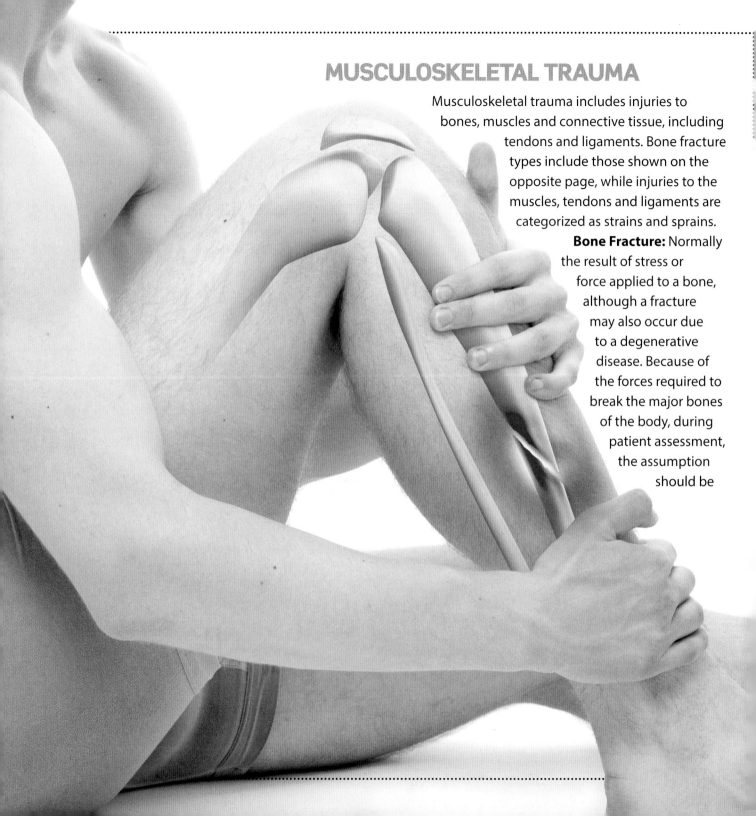

MUSCULOSKELETAL TRAUMA

Musculoskeletal trauma includes injuries to bones, muscles and connective tissue, including tendons and ligaments. Bone fracture types include those shown on the opposite page, while injuries to the muscles, tendons and ligaments are categorized as strains and sprains.

Bone Fracture: Normally the result of stress or force applied to a bone, although a fracture may also occur due to a degenerative disease. Because of the forces required to break the major bones of the body, during patient assessment, the assumption should be

MUSCULOSKELETAL TRAUMA
FRACTURE TYPES

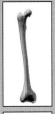

Normal Bone:
An unbroken bone will be straight, with no deformities or bumps.

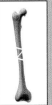

Comminuted Fracture:
Fracture involving multiple breaks in the bone, which cause bone fragment damage.

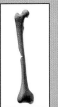

Greenstick Fracture:
Fracture in which the bone is bent but is only broken on the outside of the bend. These injuries are common in children.

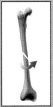

Spiral Fracture:
Fracture resulting from a twisting motion.

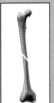

Oblique Fracture:
Fracture involving the breaking of the bone at a slanted angle.

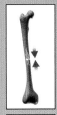

Impacted Fracture:
Fracture that occurs when one end of the bone is driven into the other.

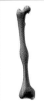

Buckle Fracture:
Also known as a "torus fracture." Characterized by a bulge in the mid-shaft of the bone, caused by an incomplete break.

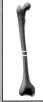

Segmental Fracture:
Fracture with two or more breaks, leaving at least one segment of bone free floating and unattached.

Transverse Fracture:
Fracture that involves the break occurring at a right angle to the long part of the bone.

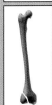

Avulsed Fracture:
When a fragment of a bone has broken away from the main mass of the bone.

made that those same forces may have damaged organs and vessels or that they may have provided a sufficient MOI to warrant spinal precautions. In addition, unless immobilized quickly, the ends of broken bones may further damage underlying muscles or blood vessels. While most bone fractures are not considered life threats, fractures of the femur and pelvis do constitute life threats due to significant blood loss, as are rib fractures due to their likelihood of damaging underlying organs.

Strain: An injury to a muscle or muscle and tendon, where it has become overextended or stretched, usually resulting from excessive physical effort.

Sprain: An injury to a joint resulting in tearing of ligaments.

Signs and Symptoms

Signs and symptoms of bone, muscle, tendon or ligament trauma include:

- A deformity or angulation
- Pain and tenderness in the affected area
- Swelling
- Bruising or other discoloration
- A grating or crunching sound/feeling as the area is palpated or as the bone moves (referred to as "crepitus")

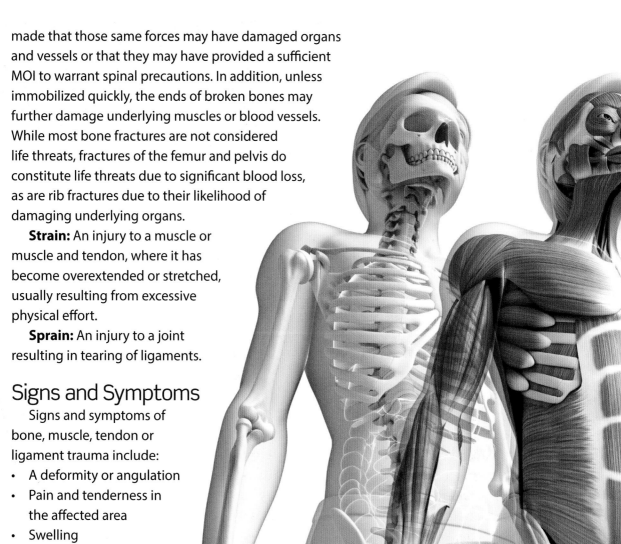

- Exposed bone ends
- Joint locked into position
- Severe weakness or loss of use of the limb
- Numbness and tingling at the affected area
- Loss of pulses distal to injury
- Cyanosis distal to injury

General Steps for Splinting the Upper and Lower Extremities

In the following section, I'll explain in detail the steps for applying nine different splints for various musculoskeletal trauma. There are a number of general steps that would apply when splinting any upper or lower extremity (other than the femur). Those steps include:

- Remove or cut away clothing to expose the injury site.
- On the affected limb, assess the patient's pulse, motor function (ask her to wiggle her fingers or toes on the injured limb) and sensation (touch a finger or toe on the injured limb and ask her to tell you which one you touched). This test is referred to as "Assessing PMS" for pulse, motor and sensation.
- Align the limb with gentle traction before splinting if any of the following are true: if the extremity lacks pulses, if it lacks motor function or sensation, if there is a severe deformity, or if the extremity distal

[**dis**-tal]
In a direction away from the center of the body and toward the extremities.

[**crep**-it-tus]
A grating or crunching sound or sensation caused by the broken ends of the bone moving over each other.

to the injury is cyanotic (a bluish color, indicating a lack of circulation and oxygen). However, if you find resistance, if there is an increase in pain or if you hear or feel crepitus, splint the extremity in the position that it was found. Generally, EMS will make one attempt to realign a limb. If that attempt is not successful, the extremity will be splinted in the position that it was found.

- Splint the extremity in a position of comfort. In most cases, the patient will already have the extremity in a position of comfort, such as cradling a broken lower arm.
- If a joint is injured, the bones above and below the injured joint should be immobilized during splinting.
- If a bone is injured, the joints above and below the injured bone should be immobilized during splinting.
- Cover any open wounds with a sterile dressing.
- Do not intentionally replace any protruding bones. Instead, cover the ends of the protruding bone with a moist, sterile dressing.
- After splinting is complete, reassess PMS. If a compromise in PMS is found, adjust the splint and re-evaluate.
- Applying ice to the affected area will reduce the pain and swelling.
- Monitor your patient for shock and arrange transport to an emergency room.

SAM Splints

Although earlier uses have been documented, the battlefield use of splinting for the treatment of musculoskeletal trauma gained in popularity during the French and Indian War (1754–1763), where field surgeons would splint broken bones by using wooden boards secured with rope, cloth or rawhide. Although World War I saw the introduction of molded plywood splints for setting leg fractures, those splints were too big and bulky to carry on the battlefield (where a broken arm or leg would more likely be splinted with broken sections from an ammunition box). During the Vietnam War, splints issued to combat medics and field surgeons were often made from inflexible plywood or cardboard and wire contraptions that wouldn't hold their shape (wet or dry). After

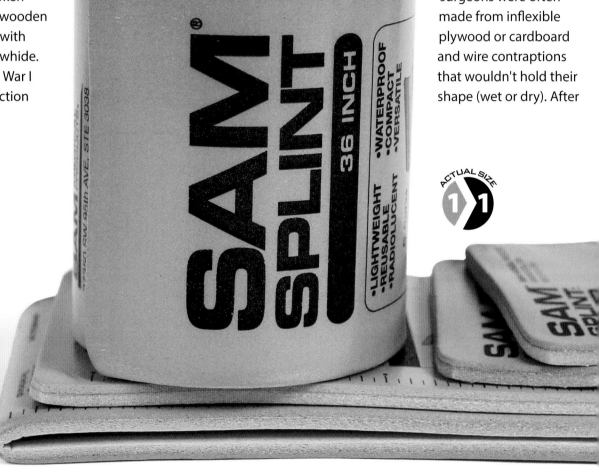

working a 24-hour shift, one of those field surgeons had a revelation after rolling a gum wrapper around his finger. That surgeon was Dr. Sam Scheinberg, who realized that although the thin aluminum foil was relatively weak and flexible when it was flat, it gained strength and rigidity when it was slightly curved. After returning to the U.S. after his tour in Vietnam, Dr. Scheinberg began experimenting with thin sheets of aluminum covered in soft, flexible foam. Dr. Scheinberg realized that even aluminum thin enough to cut with a standard scissors could be rigid enough to splint a variety of musculoskeletal trauma if the proper shape and curve were introduced. After several years working with a variety of prototypes, Dr. Scheinberg released

the first commercially available SAM Splint. Today, SAM Splints are carried by nearly every ambulance service and combat medic in the world. Since its release in 1985, SAM Medical Products has continued to create innovative emergency first-aid devices, including valved and non-valved chest seals and the SAM Pelvic Sling II, designed to stabilize a broken pelvis. While the uses of SAM Splints are almost immeasurable, I've provided step-by-step instructions on the following pages for the most common uses of the 36-inch, 18-inch, 9-inch and finger splints to splint a variety of upper and lower extremity musculoskeletal trauma, and even a field-expedient version of a cervical spine collar.

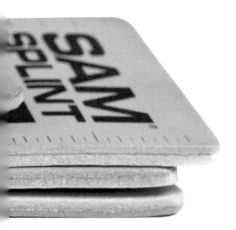

SAM Splint Sizes
SAM Splints are available in a variety of sizes but can also be cut with trauma shears or household scissors to create a splint of any size. Standard sizes are 36 inches, which are available in a flat package or in a roll, 18 inches, 9 inches and in a size perfect for finger splints.

The Science Behind SAM Splints

The science behind SAM Splints is simple: Curves are stronger than non-curves. As explained by Dr. Scheinberg, SAM splints follow the mechanics of curved surfaces. It's the same physics that lets engineers build bridges and skyscrapers out of hollow beams or I-beams rather than massive solid steel or concrete. The same physics apply to SAM splints. In its "virgin" or flat state, a SAM splint is easily molded into just about any shape, and it can even be cut with trauma shears or household

■ Virgin SAM Splint

A SAM Splint in its virgin state (without any bends) is completely malleable but offers little or no strength or support.

■ The C-Curve

To create the C-Curve, place both thumbs in the center of the SAM Splint, then pull the edges of the splint toward you to create a smooth curve. The C-curve adds strength and rigidity to the splint for a variety of uses. For greater strength, the curve can be deepened.

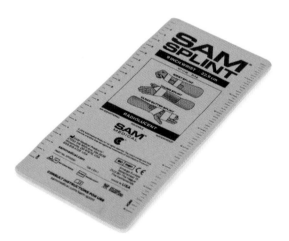

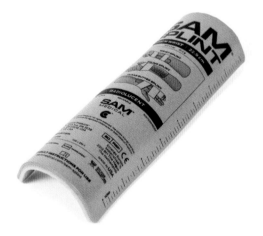

STRONG

scissors. Yet as a soon as a curve has been added, such as those shown below, the splint becomes rigid and strong enough to support a fracture of the arm, leg and even neck. Using the "Reverse C-Curve" or "T-Curve" shown below on a 36-inch SAM splint, it's even possible to make an emergency paddle, which will be nearly as rigid as an aluminum or wooden paddle. In each of the splint examples which follows, one of the first steps will be to apply one of the curves shown below.

■ The Reverse C-Curve

The Reverse C-Curve adds additional strength to the C-Curve by folding the edges of a C-Curved splint back in the reverse direction.

■ The T-Curve

To create the T-Curve, fold the splint in half along its long axis, then fold half of each side in the opposite direction to create a "T"-shaped beam. This bend adds exceptional strength to the splint and can be placed on the outside of other splints to strengthen them.

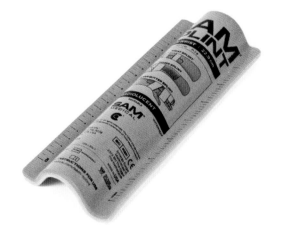

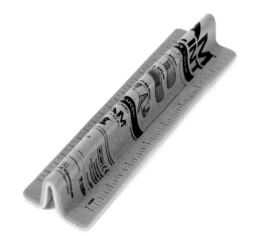

STRONGER

STRONGEST

■Volar Wrist

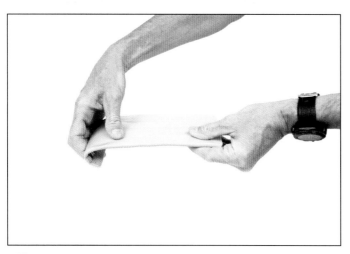

Step 1: Roll the end of a 9-inch SAM Splint over to provide a comfortable place for the fingers to rest.

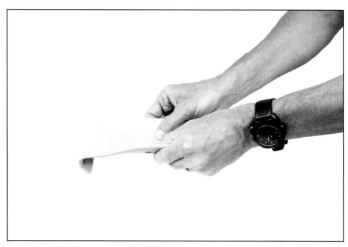

Step 2: Apply a C-Curve.

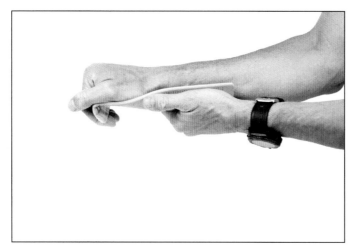

Step 3: Using your own right or left hand as a template, mold the splint into the appropriate shape for a position of comfort for the patient.

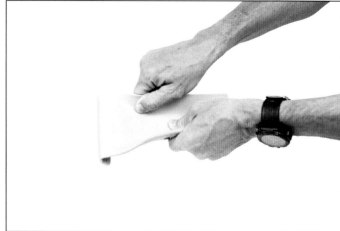

Step 4: Create a curve for the base of the thumb. Add additional strength by folding up the ulnar (little finger) side of the splint.

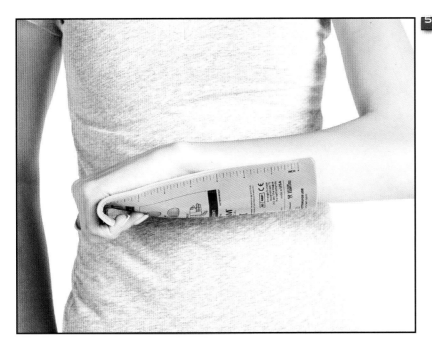

Step 5: Apply the splint to the patient and make adjustments as necessary.

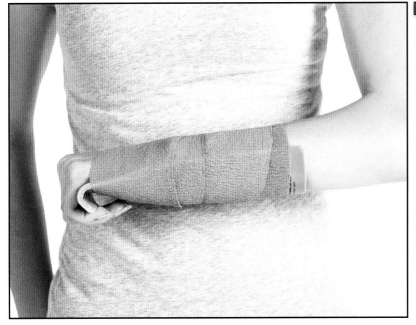

Step 6: Secure the splint with self-sticking tape, such as Coban or CoFlex.

■Thumb Spica

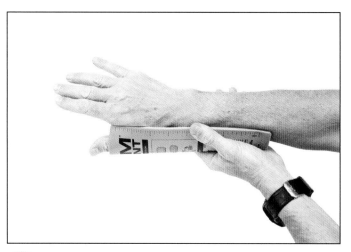

Step 1: Using your own right or left thumb and wrist as a template, mold a 9-inch SAM Splint into the thumb spica shape.

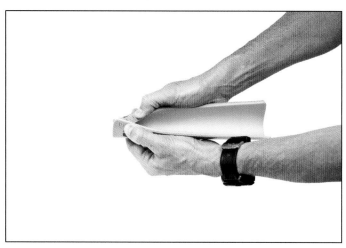

Step 2: Roll the inside edge of the splint to form a pocket for the thumb to rest.

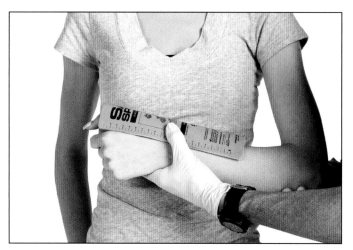

Step 3: Apply the splint to the patient and make adjustments as necessary.

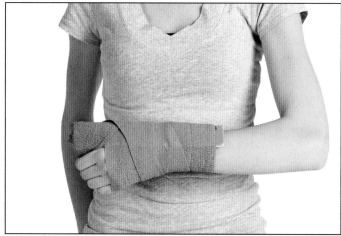

Step 4: Secure the splint with self-sticking tape, such as Coban or CoFlex.

■Ulnar Gutter

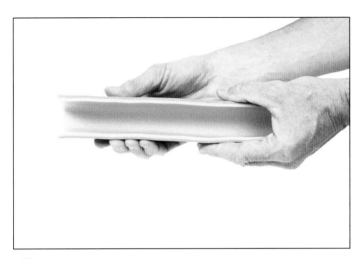

Step 1: Fold a 9-inch SAM Splint lengthwise.

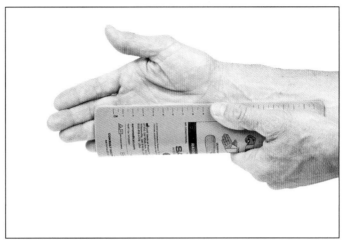

Step 2: Using the ulnar side of your own hand and wrist as a template, mold the splint into the desired shape.

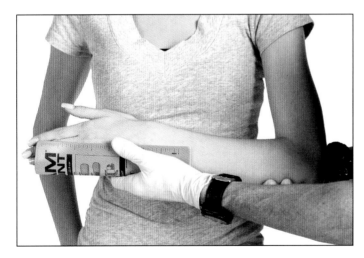

Step 3: Apply the splint to the patient and make adjustments as necessary.

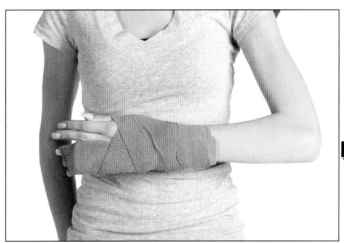

Step 4: Secure the splint with self-sticking tape, such as Coban or CoFlex.

■ Double-Layer Wrist

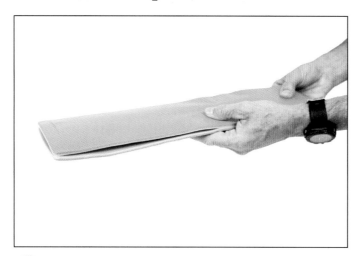

■ **Step 1:** Fold a 36-inch SAM Splint in half, end to end.

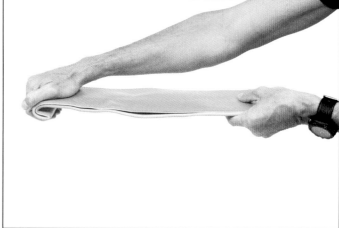

■ **Step 2:** Roll the end over to provide a comfortable place for the fingers to rest.

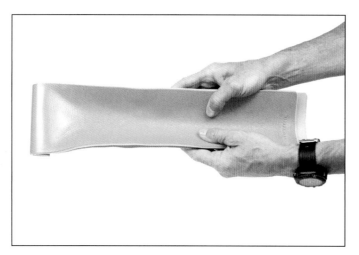

■ **Step 3:** Add strength by creating a C-Curve.

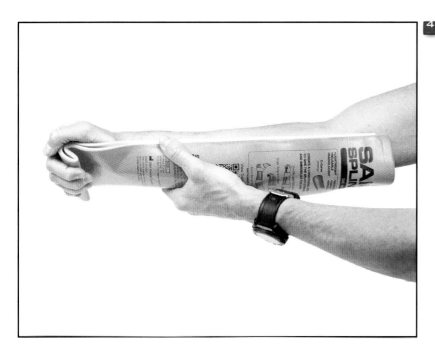

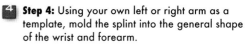

Step 4: Using your own left or right arm as a template, mold the splint into the general shape of the wrist and forearm.

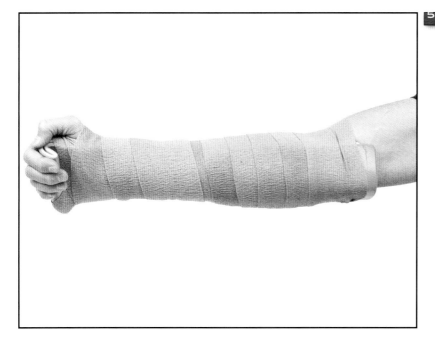

Step 5: Apply to patient and make fine adjustments as necessary. Secure the splint with self-sticking tape, such as Coban or CoFlex.

■Sugar Tong (Lower Arm)

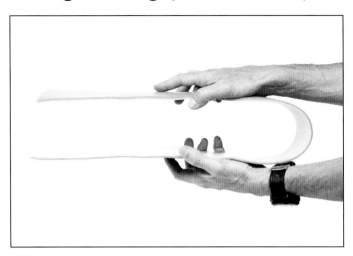

■ **Step 1:** Roll a 36-inch SAM Splint in half.

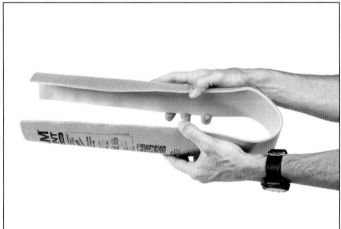

Step 2: Form a C-Curve in each half, starting from the open end of the splint and ending approximately two-thirds of the distance to the bend.

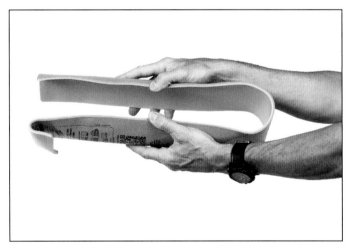

Step 3: Roll the end over to provide a comfortable place for the fingers to rest.

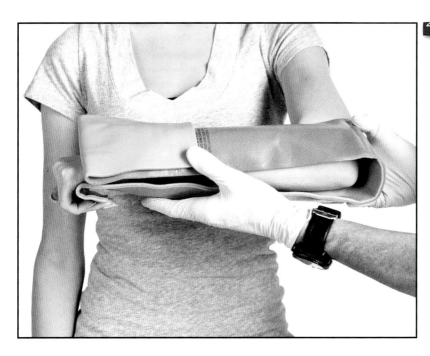

Step 4: Fit the splint to the patient. Make fine adjustments as necessary.

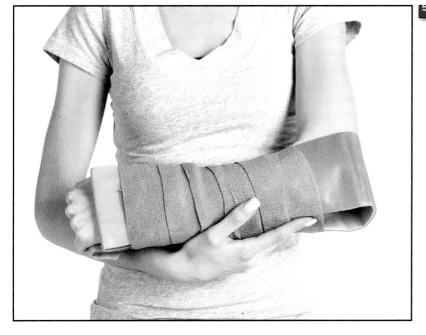

Step 5: Secure the splint with self-sticking tape, such as Coban or CoFlex. Support in a position of comfort using a triangular bandage sling.

■Humeral Shaft (Upper Arm)

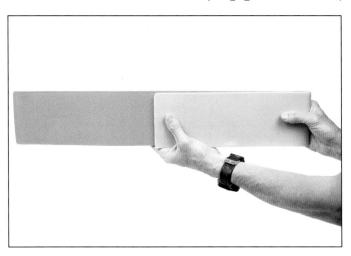

Step 1: Fold one-third of a 36-inch SAM Splint upon itself to create a 12-inch section of double-layered splint.

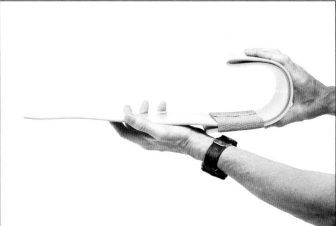

Step 2: Roll the double layer into a fishhook shape and secure the double-layer with self-sticking tape, such as Coban or CoFlex.

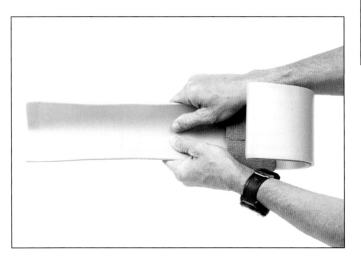

Step 3: Form a C-Curve along the shank of the fishhook for strength and fit.

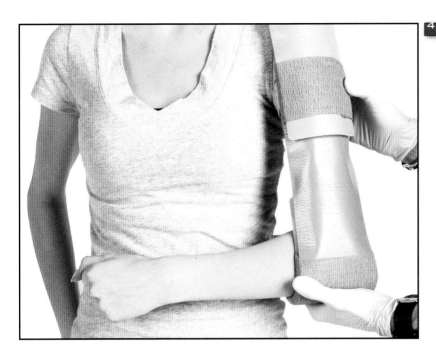

Step 4: Apply the splint to the patient. Fold any excess splint back upon itself and secure with self-sticking tape. Make fine adjustments as necessary.

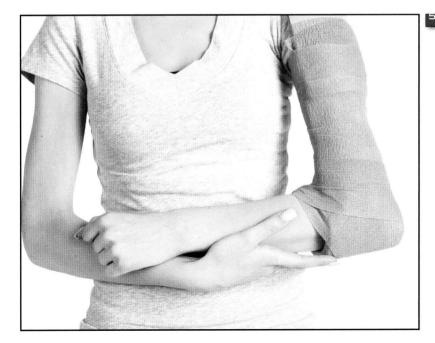

Step 5: Secure the splint with self-sticking tape, such as Coban or CoFlex. Support in a position of comfort using a triangular bandage sling.

■Cervical Collar

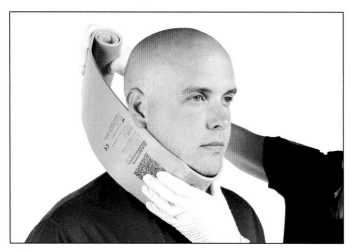

Step 1: Fold a 36-inch SAM Splint 5 inches from the end. Bracing your thumbs on each side of the fold, pull the upper edges toward you to create a V-shaped chin rest. Place the chin rest beneath the patient's chin and lower jaw. Be careful to avoid pressure on the front of the neck. Loop the remaining portion of the splint loosely around the neck.

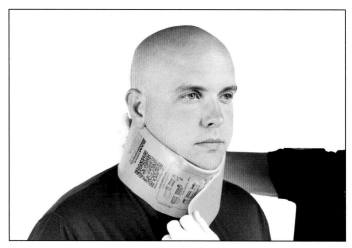

Step 2: Bring the end forward and down diagonally until it touches the chest. This creates the correct chin-to-chest distance for the chin post.

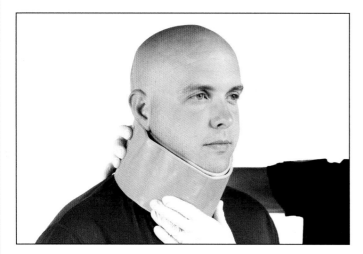

Step 3: While continuing to support the chin, bring the chest portion of the splint around the original chin rest to create a chin-post. Squeeze to deepen the chin-post.

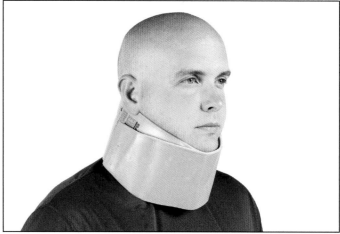

Step 4: Adjust if required by inserting your index fingers in each side of the looped splint and pulling outward to adjust. Splint may be secured with self-sticking tape, such as Coban or CoFlex.

■Finger Splint

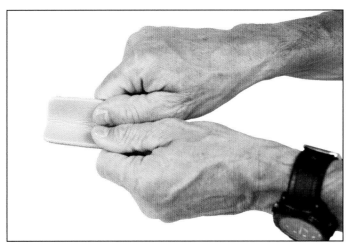

Step 1: Add a C-Curve to a SAM Finger Splint.

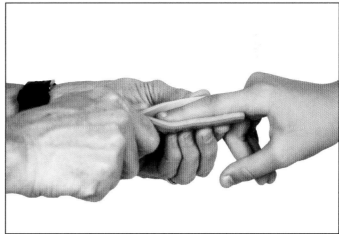

Step 2: Place the patient's injured finger into the splint and squeeze the end of the splint to create a finger guard.

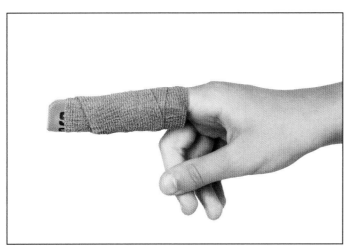

Step 3: Make fine adjustments as necessary. Secure with self-sticking tape, such as Coban or CoFlex.

■ Ankle Holster

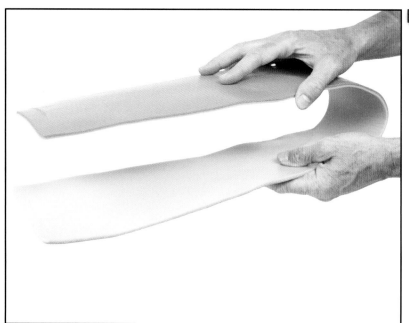

Step 1: Roll a 36-inch SAM Splint in half.

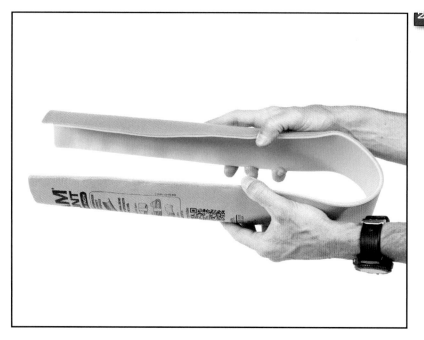

Step 2: Form a C-Curve in each half, starting from the open end of the splint and ending approximately two-thirds of the distance to the bend.

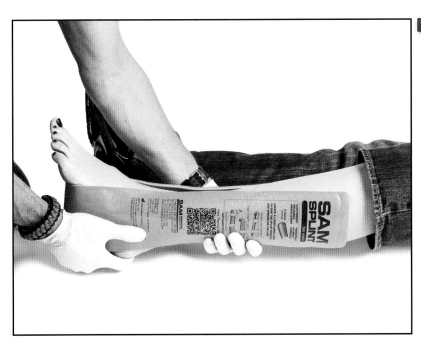

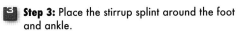 **Step 3:** Place the stirrup splint around the foot and ankle.

Step 4: Make fine adjustments as necessary. Secure with self-sticking tape, such as Coban or CoFlex.

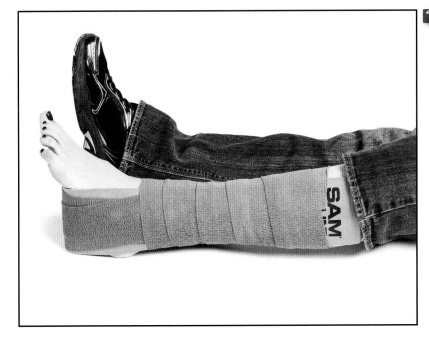

FRACTURED FEMUR

With 206 bones in our body, most of us don't make it past adolescence without breaking at least one of them. Although the typical broken bone might cause significant pain, most broken bones wouldn't be categorized as significant life threats. But that isn't the case with a broken femur or broken pelvis. Both the femur and pelvis bones contain large blood vessels that, when broken, can leak and cause a large amount of blood to be lost internally. For example, a broken femur can easily cause a patient to lose 1.5 liters of blood (almost a third of the average adult's total volume), while a broken pelvis can cause as much as 2 liters of blood to be lost into the pelvic cavity. As you'd suspect, both injuries are extremely serious, and your patient needs immediate evacuation to a trauma center. You can rank these injuries right up there with a sucking chest wound. If you are hours or days away from rescue, you'll need to stabilize your patient's injuries to the best of your ability.

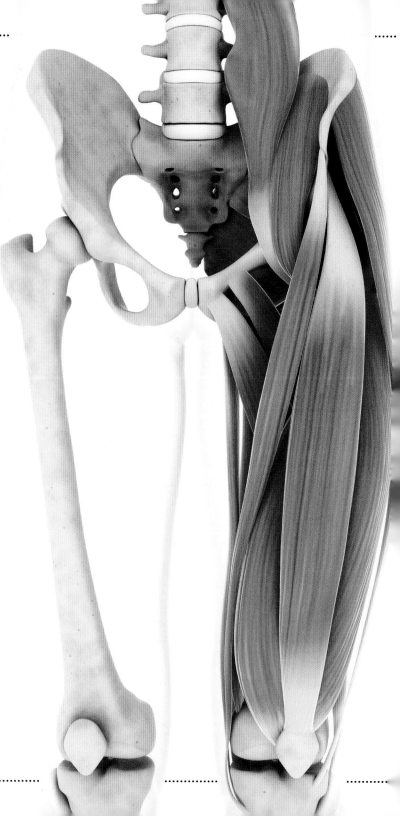

Fractured Femur
The average adult male femur is approximately 19 inches long and 0.9 inches in diameter. When a femur is fractured, it can cause a patient to lose as much as one-third of his or her total blood volume. In addition, after the femur has fractured, the powerful leg muscles will contract, causing the broken ends of the bone to slide past one another, causing additional damage to underlying muscle and vessels and creating a large cavity where blood can continue to pool.

Signs and Symptoms

In addition to your patient's agonized screams, a good indicator of a broken femur will be if the patient's upper leg seems to have shortened or seems to have grown another knee. Shortening of the leg may occur because the muscles of the upper leg are under significant tension, and when the femur breaks, the tension of the muscles pulls the broken edges of the bones over one another (this overlap will appear as a bulge or a "second knee" on the leg). The contraction of the leg muscles will not only cause an amazing amount of pain but also damage the vessels running through and around the femur. It creates a large cavity in which blood can continue to be lost. Unlike other splinting techniques, which are designed to simply hold a broken bone in a position of comfort, a special type of splint, referred to as a "traction splint," is required for a femur break. A traction splint is designed to counteract the contraction of the thigh muscles by providing 10-15 pounds of pressure (or more) in the opposite direction of the contraction. An ankle cuff and a rigid frame work to either push or pull the foot in a direction opposite the contraction.

While most ambulances carry large commercial splints, there are now a number of portable traction splints suitable for a large emergency first-aid kit (including the ski-pole/hiking-pole traction splint demonstrated in the next section), and a number of simple, field-expedient methods are available. However, for a traction splint to be considered for use, the femur break must be a midline break, which may present itself as a large lump on the midline of the femur. A number of contraindications (reasons why you wouldn't use a particular treatment) also exist.

CONTRAINDICATION

[contra-indi-**k**-shun]
A specific situation or set of criteria in which a procedure or drug should not be used because it may be harmful to the patient.

Those contraindications include:

- The femur is broken within 2 inches of the knee or the pelvis.
- The knee is broken or injured.
- A bone of the lower leg is broken.
- The ankle is broken or injured.
- The pelvis is broken. This can be determined by gently pressing on both sides of the pelvis bone, feeling for stability. If the pelvis feels unstable, it is most likely broken, and a traction splint should not be used.
- The broken femur bone is protruding through the skin.
- In addition to the broken femur, the upper or lower leg is partially amputated.

If none of the contraindications exist, you can immediately provide manual traction on the broken leg by placing a rescuer at the patient's feet and having the rescuer grasp the patient's foot or ankle, pulling with enough tension on the leg so that it reverts back to its normal length (or close to its normal length). In most cases, the patient will have an immediate reduction in pain. While a rescuer can hold manual stabilization for a short period of time, that person can easily become fatigued while pulling against the tension of the large leg muscles, and a commercial or field-expedient traction splint may be required to continue to hold tension while waiting for EMS. If any of the contraindications do exist, or if the patient is also suffering from other trauma (including other broken bones), the simplest and most effective way to treat the patient is to immobilize their entire body on a long board or a field-expedient substitute. The reality is, the forces required to break a femur are so significant that it is highly likely that your patient will be suffering from multiple traumatic injuries, which means that full immobilization, rapid transport (which may include air evacuation) and treatment for shock may be the only treatments that are available to you.

Providing Manual Traction

If none of the contraindications exist, you can immediately provide manual traction on the broken leg by placing a rescuer at the patient's feet and having the rescuer grasp the patient's foot or ankle, pulling with enough tension on the leg so that it reverts back to its normal length (or close to its normal length). While this may sound like torture, in most cases, the patient will have an *immediate* reduction in pain.

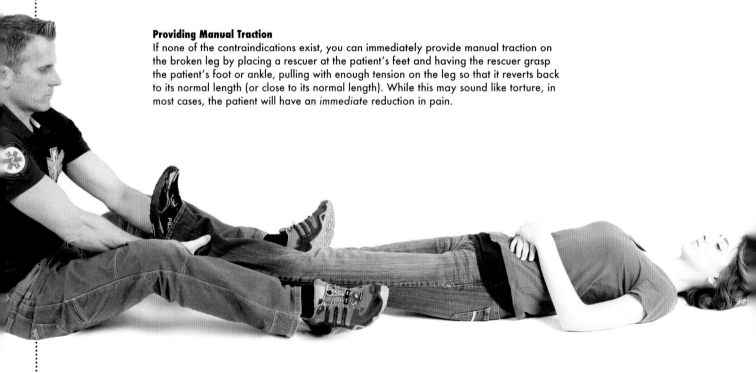

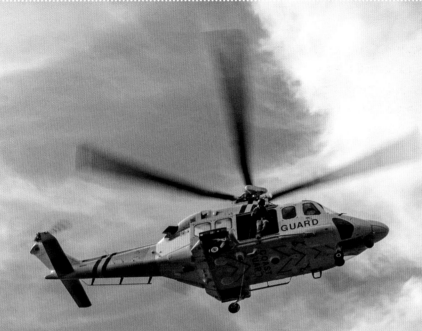

There are a number of traumatic emergencies that must receive immediate evacuation to a trauma center, which may include evacuation by air transport.

Commercial Traction Splint

First developed by Welsh surgeon Hugh Owen Thomas and put into use during World War I, the traction splint is now standard equipment on ambulances and at battlefield aid stations around the world. The two most common commercial traction splints in use today — the Sagar and Hare traction splints — lack the portability to fit into the average field trauma bag, yet a number of new, commercially available traction splints are both effective and

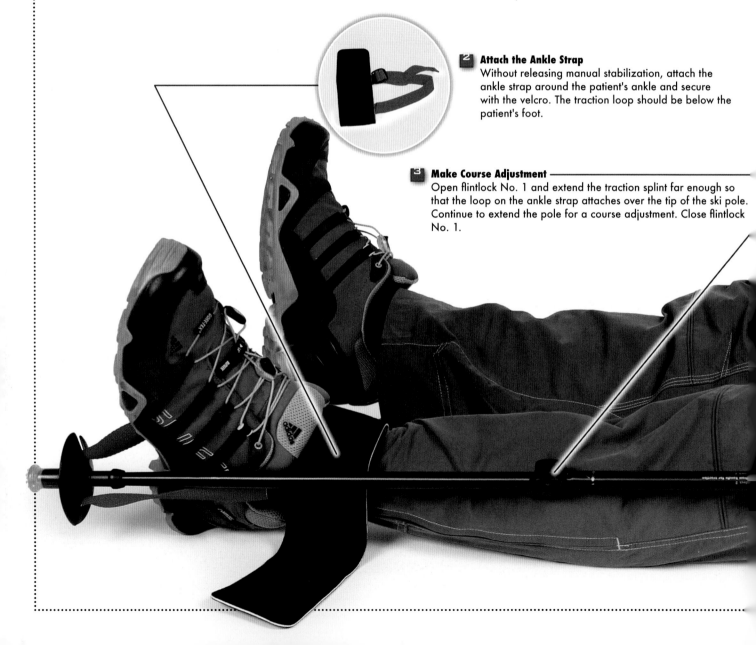

2 Attach the Ankle Strap
Without releasing manual stabilization, attach the ankle strap around the patient's ankle and secure with the velcro. The traction loop should be below the patient's foot.

3 Make Course Adjustment
Open flintlock No. 1 and extend the traction splint far enough so that the loop on the ankle strap attaches over the tip of the ski pole. Continue to extend the pole for a course adjustment. Close flintlock No. 1.

portable, including the Kendrick Traction Device (KTD) and the Slishman Traction Splint (STS), which is available as a standard splint or in the innovative ski-/hiking-pole model shown here. The model below ships with two ski/hiking poles, one of which is a standard pole and the other which is designed to convert into a traction splint within one to two minutes. To apply the STS, follow the step-by-step instructions below. Note that the steps should be read in numeric order, not left to right.

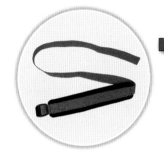

Attach the Groin Strap

After one rescuer takes manual stabilization of the femur, a second rescuer should attach the groin strap around the patient's upper thigh. It should be tightened so that two fingers can still fit between it and the patient's leg. Attach the groin strap through the hand strap on the ski-pole traction splint or connect with a carabiner.

4 Apply Traction

Open flintlock No. 2 and pull the cord at the top of the ski pole to apply traction. When the leg has returned to the same length (or close to the same length) as the uninjured leg, close flintlock No. 2.

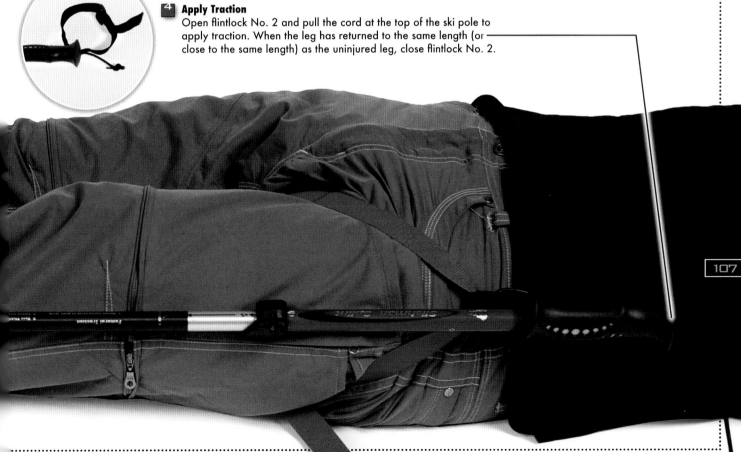

Field-Expedient Traction Splint

While a commercial traction splint might be preferable to a field-expedient traction splint, the reality is that a field-expedient splint can be created in just minutes using common items that would be found on a typical camping, hiking, hunting or canoe trip, including webbing or rope, carabiners and a rigid item (such as a ski or hiking pole, a paddle or a solid branch). While you might have your doubts about the effectiveness of a field-expedient traction splint versus a commercially available splint, a study by the Wilderness and Environmental Medicine Society tested

Gather Supplies

Collect the supplies needed to make the field-expedient traction splint, including a ski or hiking pole, three carabiniers, 550 cord and at least 6 feet of nylon webbing.

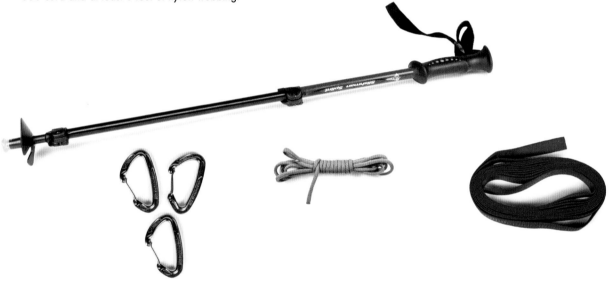

A Part A: The Ankle Strap

Using a 3-foot length of webbing, form it into a loop and tie an overhand knot with each end back onto the standing part of the webbing on the opposite side of the loop (this is referred to as a "fisherman's knot"). This will create an adjustable opening between the two knots for the ankle and a loop on the bottom that will be used to pull traction. Attach a carabiner to the bottom loop.

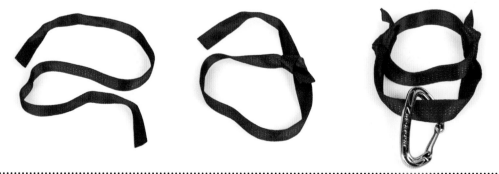

three commercially available splints side-by-side against a field-expedient splint using 10 test subjects. After a 30-minute application of each option, the researchers found no measurable difference in the pounds of force generated (which ranged from 10.4-13.3 pounds), the comfort or the stability of the commercial splints versus the field-expedient splint. To create a field-expedient traction splint similar to the one tested by WMS, follow the step-by-step instructions below to create the individual parts, A-D. These parts will be used to construct the field-expedient traction splint as shown on the following two pages.

 Part B: Groin Strap
Using a 3-foot length of webbing, tie an overhand knot at the end and attach a carabiner.

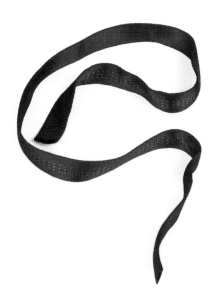

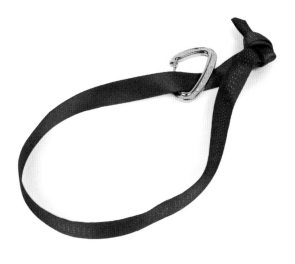

 Part C: Standing End of Pulley System
With a 12-inch piece of 550 cord, tie a Figure 8 on a bight at each end. Attach a carabiner to one end.

 Part D: Work End of Pulley System
With a 3- to 4-foot piece of 550 cord, tie a Figure 8 on a bight on one end.

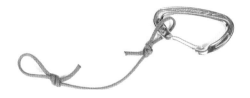

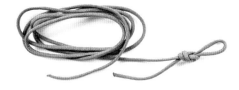

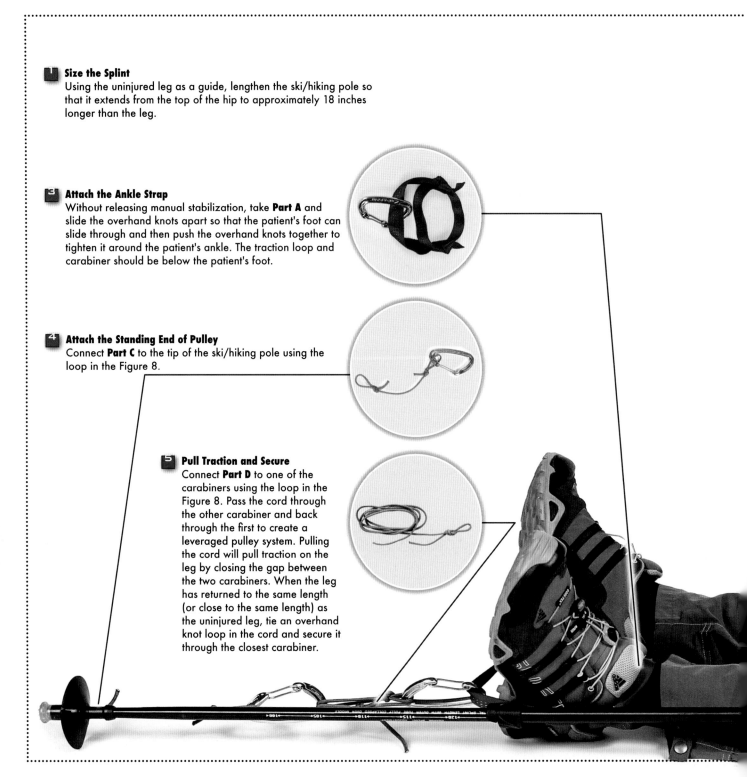

Size the Splint

Using the uninjured leg as a guide, lengthen the ski/hiking pole so that it extends from the top of the hip to approximately 18 inches longer than the leg.

Attach the Ankle Strap

Without releasing manual stabilization, take **Part A** and slide the overhand knots apart so that the patient's foot can slide through and then push the overhand knots together to tighten it around the patient's ankle. The traction loop and carabiner should be below the patient's foot.

Attach the Standing End of Pulley

Connect **Part C** to the tip of the ski/hiking pole using the loop in the Figure 8.

Pull Traction and Secure

Connect **Part D** to one of the carabiners using the loop in the Figure 8. Pass the cord through the other carabiner and back through the first to create a leveraged pulley system. Pulling the cord will pull traction on the leg by closing the gap between the two carabiners. When the leg has returned to the same length (or close to the same length) as the uninjured leg, tie an overhand knot loop in the cord and secure it through the closest carabiner.

2 Attach the Groin Strap

After one rescuer takes manual stabilization of the femur, a second rescuer should attach **Part B** around the patient's upper thigh. Attach the groin strap through the hand strap on the ski/hiking pole using the carabiner.

If webbing is not available, the groin strap may be created using a camera strap or a belt.

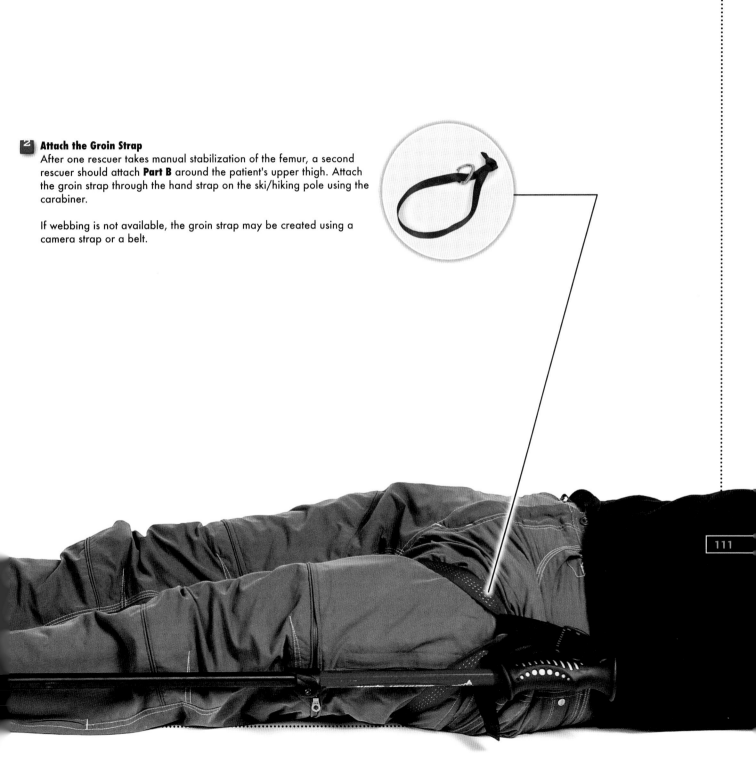

PELVIS FRACTURES

The pelvis is a donut-shaped ring of fused bones that connects the upper and lower skeleton and is designed to hold the weight of the upper body and protect organs housed in the lower abdominal cavity, including the bladder; the urethra; the end of the large intestine and the internal reproductive organs; and major blood vessels, including the iliac arteries (which feed the femoral arteries) and the iliac veins (which return blood from the extremities).

The ilium make up the wings of the pelvis, which are connected in the back (the posterior) by the sacrum and coccyx (the bottom two bones of the spine) and in front by the symphysis pubis. As with a fractured femur or fractured ribs, a fractured pelvis can also lead to severe blood loss as the fractured

Sacroiliac Joint
Joins the Iliac Crest with the Sacrum. Common location for fracture.

Sacrum
The bottom of the spine, which forms the back wall of the pelvic ring.

Ischium
When you stand, your weight is supported by the pelvic ring. When you sit, your weight is supported by the ischium.

ends of the bone damage the iliac arteries and veins. It can also damage the organs contained within the pelvic girdle. Pelvic fractures can range from simple to complex. A fracture to the upper wing of the ilium (known as the iliac crest) can cause significant pain and tenderness, but it's unlikely to damage organs or vessels. A fracture of the pelvic ring, however, must be considered a significant life threat. In fact, uncontrolled bleeding is the No. 1 cause of death for patients with a complex pelvic fracture. A pelvic ring fracture can occur in any of the locations where the separate bones are fused together, such as between the sacrum and ilium or between the two pubis bones. The pelvis ring may also fracture in multiple locations. Pelvic ring fractures are often referred to as "open book" fractures because the previously closed and stable pelvic ring is now open.

Iliac Crests
Will fracture if sufficient force is applied, but typically would not constitute a life threat.

Ilium
Form the wings of the pelvic ring.

Pubis
Forms the front wall of the pelvic ring.

Symphysis Pubis
Joins the left and right ilium in the front of the pelvic ring.

Signs and Symptoms:

- A significant mechanism of injury has occurred (such as a fall from a significant height for a younger patient or from a standing height or higher for an elderly patient), and the patient complains of hip or pelvic pain, lower extremity numbness and tingling, or lower-back pain.
- A rapid trauma assessment has uncovered instability, deformities, movement of bones that should be stable or crepitus. To conduct this assessment, use the palms of your hands to gently push inward and then downward on the iliac crests and then downward on the pubis bones.

Like the field treatment for a broken femur or flail chest, the splinting of a fractured pelvis is different than the type of splinting required for an upper extremity or lower-leg fracture, strain or sprain.

Field Treatment

When EMS is more than an hour away, the fractured pelvis can be stabilized by folding a standard-sized sheet lengthwise into a 12-inch-wide swathe. With the assistance of additional rescuers, slide the swathe under the patient and tie it using an overhand knot. Do not overtighten. For a commercial version of a pelvic sling, see Chapter 4.

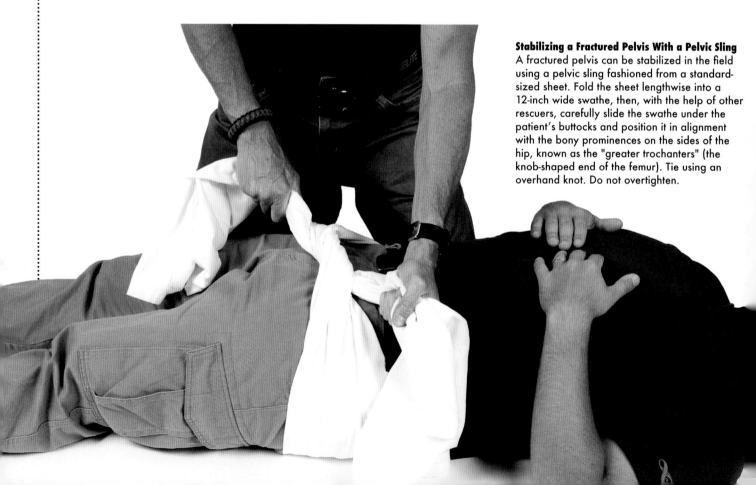

Stabilizing a Fractured Pelvis With a Pelvic Sling
A fractured pelvis can be stabilized in the field using a pelvic sling fashioned from a standard-sized sheet. Fold the sheet lengthwise into a 12-inch wide swathe, then, with the help of other rescuers, carefully slide the swathe under the patient's buttocks and position it in alignment with the bony prominences on the sides of the hip, known as the "greater trochanters" (the knob-shaped end of the femur). Tie using an overhand knot. Do not overtighten.

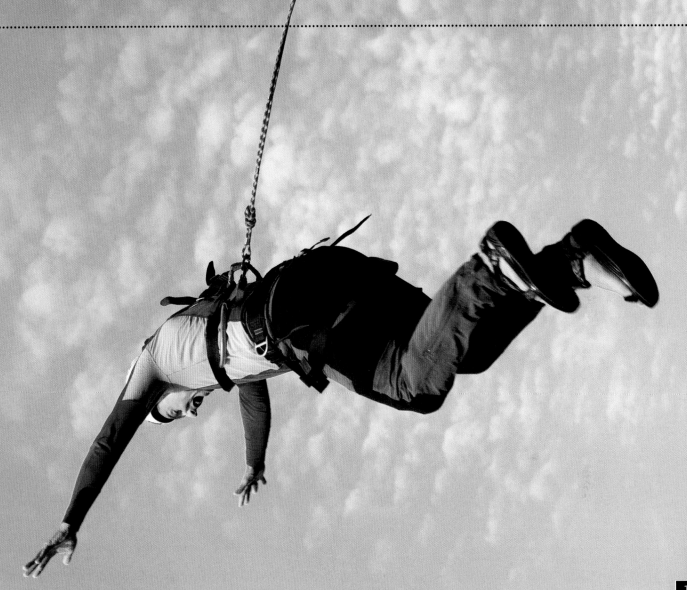

■ A fall from a cliff, a ladder or even a standing height (for an elderly patient) risks a pelvis fracture. After any significant MOI, assess the pelvis for stability, deformities or crepitus during the rapid trauma assessment.

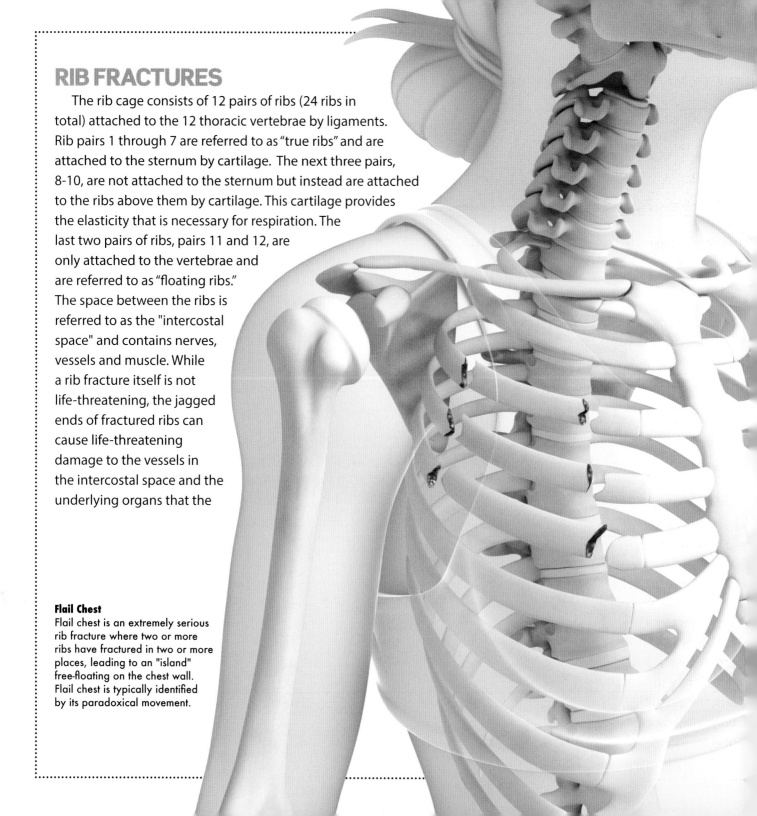

RIB FRACTURES

The rib cage consists of 12 pairs of ribs (24 ribs in total) attached to the 12 thoracic vertebrae by ligaments. Rib pairs 1 through 7 are referred to as "true ribs" and are attached to the sternum by cartilage. The next three pairs, 8-10, are not attached to the sternum but instead are attached to the ribs above them by cartilage. This cartilage provides the elasticity that is necessary for respiration. The last two pairs of ribs, pairs 11 and 12, are only attached to the vertebrae and are referred to as "floating ribs." The space between the ribs is referred to as the "intercostal space" and contains nerves, vessels and muscle. While a rib fracture itself is not life-threatening, the jagged ends of fractured ribs can cause life-threatening damage to the vessels in the intercostal space and the underlying organs that the

Flail Chest

Flail chest is an extremely serious rib fracture where two or more ribs have fractured in two or more places, leading to an "island" free-floating on the chest wall. Flail chest is typically identified by its paradoxical movement.

PARADOXICAL MOVEMENT

[pair-a-**dock**-sick-all]
Movement that is the opposite of what is expected; the chest moving in rather than out on inspiration.

rib cage is meant to protect, including puncturing the lungs, leading to a closed pneumothorax.

Signs and Symptoms

- Excruciating pain with coughing, breathing, or movement
- Deformity of the chest wall
- Rapid, shallow breathing and/or difficulty breathing because of the associated pain
- Crepitation upon breathing or palpation
- Tenderness
- Guarding (holding an arm over the injured area)

Rib fractures often go unnoticed by the patient until they progressively deteriorate. In fact, the patient's only complaint may be shortness of breath (what EMS refers to as SOB). But, based upon the mechanism of injury, you must have a high degree of suspicion that trauma to the chest has occurred, and you should proceed with that assumption during your patient assessment. The most common MOIs associated with rib fractures are motor vehicle accidents, falls and assault.

Field Treatment

For a simple rib fracture, it is sufficient to splint the patient's arm over the injured area with a triangular bandage sling and a swathe. Because of the possibility of internal vessel and organ damage, early recognition and early transport is critical. As mentioned, simple rib fractures are not typically life-threatening, but that is not the case with flail chest.

Flail Chest

Flail chest is defined as two or more ribs broken in two or more places. Beyond that technical definition, flail chest results in a segment of ribs floating separately from the rest of the rib cage and chest wall. Because of the mechanics of breathing, this segment is often recognized by what's referred to as "**paradoxical movement**,"

Stabilizing Fractured Ribs
Simple fractures to the ribs can be stabilized by using a triangular bandage to splint the arm on the injured side over the fractured ribs, secured in place with a second triangular bandage fashioned into a swathe.

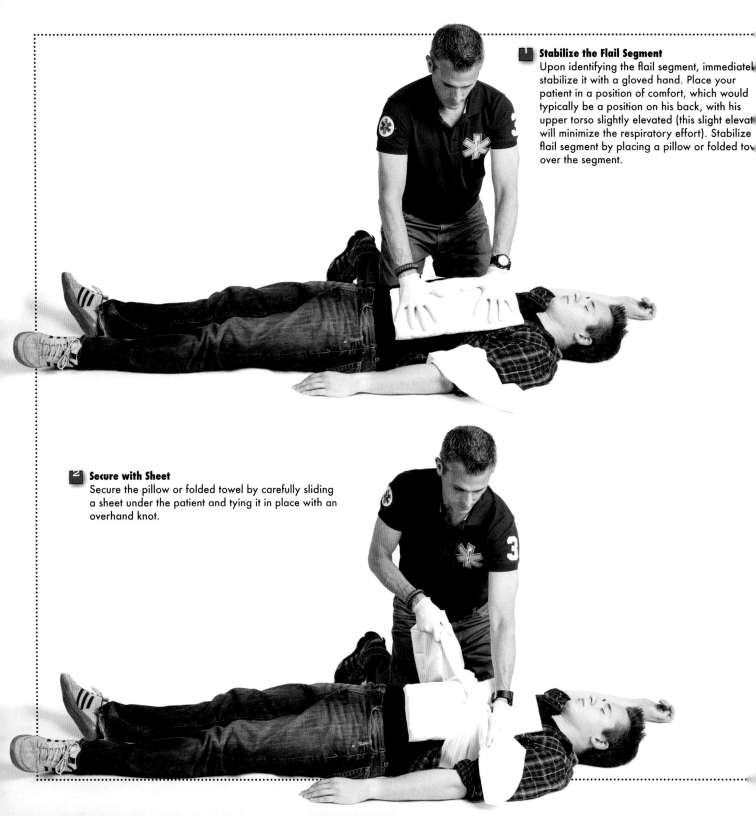

Stabilize the Flail Segment

Upon identifying the flail segment, immediate[ly] stabilize it with a gloved hand. Place your patient in a position of comfort, which would typically be a position on his back, with his upper torso slightly elevated (this slight elevat[ion] will minimize the respiratory effort). Stabilize [the] flail segment by placing a pillow or folded tov[el] over the segment.

Secure with Sheet

Secure the pillow or folded towel by carefully sliding a sheet under the patient and tying it in place with an overhand knot.

which is the flail segment moving in the opposite direction than the rest of the rib cage. In other words, when the patient breathes in and the chest wall expands, the flail segment will move in, and when the patient breathes out (and the chest contracts), the flail segment will move out. The dangers of flail chest are twofold: First, flail chest is *extremely* painful, and it will typically result in the patient taking very shallow breaths, resulting in an inadequate tidal volume (that is, air will not reach the alveoli at the base of the lungs). Since the chest wall can no longer contribute to breathing effort, patients can become exhausted very quickly. More importantly, the paradoxical movement and jagged rib edges can injure the lungs, resulting in what's referred to as a "pulmonary contusion," which will interfere with the lung's ability to effectively off-load carbon dioxide and move oxygen into the blood stream.

Signs and Symptoms

- Signs and symptoms of a rib fracture, plus paradoxical movement of a portion of the chest wall.

Flail chest is an extremely serious injury requiring emergency room care as quickly as possible. If you are miles from EMS support and your only option is to evacuate on foot, this is the type of situation where EMS should be brought to the patient rather than the patient brought to EMS. If EMS can't be reached by cellphone, keep your patient in a position of comfort and send a runner to go find help quickly.

FLAIL CHEST
EMERGENCY CARE

Here's what you should do if you find yourself with a patient who has sustained flail chest:

- Upon identifying the flail segment, immediately stabilize it with a gloved hand.
- Place your patient in a position of comfort, which would typically be a position on his or her back, with the upper torso slightly elevated. This slight elevation will minimize the respiratory effort.
- Stabilize the flail segment by placing a pillow or folded towel over the segment and secure it in place by wrapping gauze or a sheet around the patient's torso. This stabilization can minimize the paradoxical movement and help protect the lung from injury.
- If you determine that your patient's breathing rate or volume is inadequate to support his or her life, you'll need to be prepared to assist his or her breathing through artificial means.

HEAD TRAUMA

Head trauma should be considered one of the most serious conditions that can occur, particularly when outside of the umbrella of EMS. It can include trauma to the skull, the brain, the scalp and the face.

Trauma to the Skull

The skull is made up of 22 bones, including eight cranial bones that are fused together to protect the brain and 14 facial bones, including the jaw, nose, cheek and orbital socket of the eye. While any fracture of the cranial or facial bones is serious, a fracture of the temporal bone, the occipital bone or the sphenoid bone constitute what's referred to as a "**basilar skull fracture**." A fracture of these bones can damage or tear the meninges (a three-layered membrane protecting the brain), resulting in the loss of cerebrospinal fluid, which cushions and protects the brain and spinal cord. Signs and symptoms of a basilar skull fracture include:

- Clear fluid leaking from the ears or nose.
- Continuous bleeding from the ears.
- Bruising behind the ears (referred to as "battle sign").

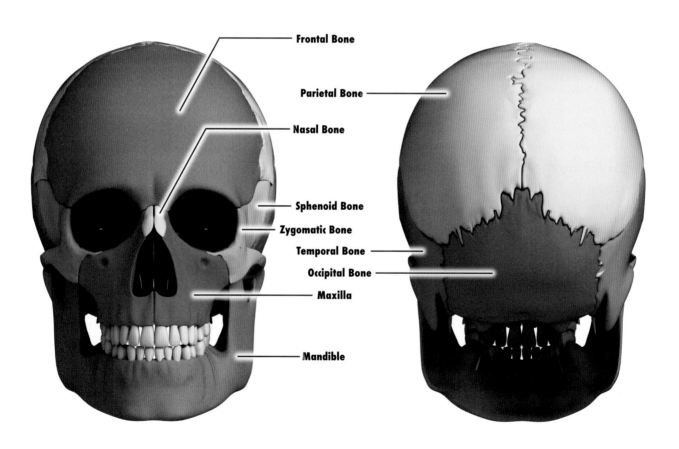

Frontal Bone

Parietal Bone

Nasal Bone

Sphenoid Bone

Zygomatic Bone

Temporal Bone

Occipital Bone

Maxilla

Mandible

Trauma to the Brain
Moderate Traumatic Brain Injury

Concussion: Considered a mild to moderate traumatic brain injury (although don't let that categorization fool you; a concussion is a serious injury requiring immediate medical evaluation), a concussion occurs when there has been sufficient force applied to the head to cause brain tissue to stretch, tear or shear. Signs and symptoms include:

- Nausea and vomiting
- Loss of memory of the incident
- Confusion or combativeness

Signs and symptoms of a concussion typically resolve within minutes of the incident. If signs and symptoms do not diminish, or if they become more pronounced, this is a sign of a more significant brain injury.

Significant Traumatic Brain Injury

Contusion: A brain contusion can occur in combination with a concussion and includes bruising, swelling or bleeding of the brain. Signs and symptoms include:

- Unequal pupils
- Decreased responsiveness
- A change in vital signs, including heart and respiratory rates

Subdural Hematoma: A subdural hematoma is a collection of blood between the outer layer and the middle layer of the meninges. Signs and symptoms include:

- Seizures
- Paralysis to one side of the body
- Dilation of one pupil
- Decreased pulse rate and respiratory rate
- Vomiting

Subdural hematomas account for about 33 percent of all serious head injuries.

Epidural Hematoma: An epidural hematoma is a pooling of blood between the outer layer of the meninges and the skull (in two-thirds of the cases, this is caused by severe arterial bleeding), which dramatically and rapidly increases intracranial pressure. Signs and symptoms can match those of a subdural hematoma, yet the epidural hematoma is a much more serious brain injury.

Trauma to the Head
Trauma to the head can include fractures to the bones of the skull; laceration to skin, muscle and underlying vessels; or concussion, contusion, hematoma, laceration or herniation of the brain.

Field Treatment

As with stroke, there is no field treatment for skull fractures or brain trauma other than early recognition, implementation of spinal cord precautions and constant monitoring of the patient's airway. Needless to say, any of these injuries are *extremely* serious and require immediate evacuation to a trauma center.

Trauma to the Scalp

The scalp has a rich supply of blood vessels that will bleed profusely when cut. Unlike vessels throughout the rest of the body, the vessels of the scalp have a limited ability to constrict when cut, and they may continue to bleed heavily and for a longer duration than for similar lacerations on another part of the body. Treatment for a scalp laceration will include direct pressure, but any time an injury to the scalp has occurred, you must consider if the MOI was significant enough to have also caused a skull fracture. For this reason, the amount of direct pressure that should be applied to a scalp laceration should not be the same as for

Field Treatment for Scalp Laceration
Compression bandages, such as the emergency bandage and "H" bandage, are perfect choices for the treatment of a lacerated scalp, but if there exists the possibility that a skull fracture has also occurred, you should not apply the full amount of pressure that can be applied. Instead, simply wrap the bandage around the injury site, layering the elastisized bandage over the pressure plate without looping through the plate and reversing direction.

lacerations on other parts of the body. If you're using a pressure bandage (such as an emergency bandage or "H" bandage), you should place the sterile dressing on the injury and wrap the elasticized bandage around the injury without wrapping the bandage through the pressure plate. The pressure applied by the elastic properties of the bandage will typically be enough pressure to slow and stop the bleed.

Trauma to the Face

Any time trauma has occurred to the face, a primary concern will be ensuring that the patient maintains a patent airway. For lacerations, avulsions (a portion of the skin has torn away) or punctures, gently apply pressure with sterile gauze or a surgical sponge and monitor the patient's airway. If the patient is not responsive, maintain an open airway with the jaw-thrust technique and examine the airway for any sign of a blockage, including blood or broken teeth.

HEAD TRAUMA
EMERGENCY CARE

Here's what you should do if you find yourself with a patient who has sustained serious head trauma:

- Determine if spinal precautions are warranted.
- If the patient is unresponsive, open the airway using the jaw-thrust method and look for any sign of blockage, such as blood or broken teeth.
- As part of your primary assessment, assess the patient for signs and symptoms of brain trauma.

Bleeding Control:

- Do not apply pressure to an open or depressed injury to the skull. Doing so can push bone fragments into the brain.
- Do not attempt to stop the flow of cerebrospinal fluid flowing from the ears. Instead, carefully cover or wrap the ears with loose sterile gauze.
- For other lacerations, apply gentle direct pressure with sterile gauze or a surgical sponge.
- If a compression bandage is used for a scalp injury, apply it without looping the bandage through the pressure plate.

TRAUMA TO THE EYE

While a serious injury to the eye wouldn't normally be considered a life threat, it would certainly be considered a quality-of-life threat and should be considered a very serious condition, depending upon its severity. Trauma to the eye can include impaled objects, damage to the globe (the eyeball itself), extruded eyeballs, fractured orbits (the bony sockets surrounding the eye) and chemical burns. Field treatment for each condition should be considered as nothing more than the required steps to minimize the damage or to protect the eye from further damage while the patient is being transported to emergency care.

Orbit
The orbit or orbital is made up of seven separate bones that encase the eyeball (the globe).

Globe
The globe is the actual eyeball encased within the orbit. The globe is typically about 1 inch in diameter and is composed of the sclera (the tough outer coating or "white" of the eye), the cornea (the clear portion of the eye covering the iris and pupil), the iris (the colored part of the eye) and the pupil (the opening that expands or contracts and allows light to enter through the lens, which is just behind the pupil).

Peri-Orbital Skin
The skin covering the orbit and surrounding the globe, including the eyelids.

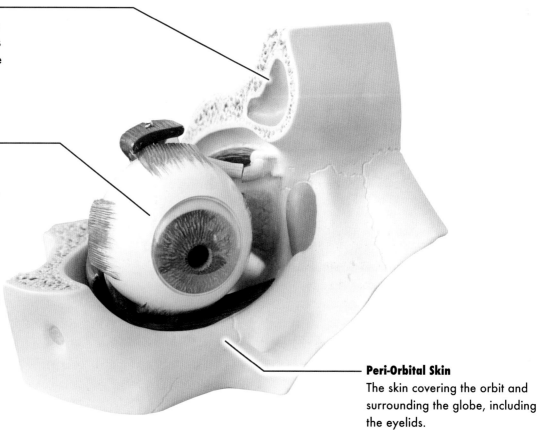

Fractured Orbit

While most of us have experienced a black eye or two in our lives, a more significant impact or mechanism of injury can fracture the bones surrounding the eyeball, known as the "orbit" or "orbital." Made up of seven small bones, the orbital bones are strong yet will fracture if the right amount of force is applied. Signs and symptoms of an orbital bone fracture include:

- A deformity upon palpation, which will be a noticeable unevenness in the normally smooth surface of the orbit
- Significant tenderness upon palpation
- Double vision, known as diplopia
- A feeling of paralysis at or around the eyebrow
- An inability for the patient to follow your finger upward

Field Treatment

- If damage to the globe is not suspected, the area surrounding the eye may be treated with ice packs to reduce swelling.
- Since significant force is required to fracture the orbital bones, spinal precautions should be taken, including taking manual stabilization of the spine.
- Arrange immediate transport to a trauma center.

Injury to the Globe

Injuries to the globe can range from foreign objects (such as dirt or an insect) on the cornea or trapped behind the eyelids to impaled objects to lacerations or deformities. I'll review the treatment for those one at a time.

Field Treatment for Foreign Object

Foreign objects in the eye that have not penetrated the globe will normally be flushed from the eye by the normal flow of tears, but if that has not occurred, the object may be removed by flushing the eye with clean water while holding the eyelid open. Ensure that the patient's head is tilted in an appropriate direction so that the foreign object doesn't get flushed from one eye and into the other eye.

If flushing the eye does not work, the foreign object may be removed using sterile gauze or a sterile swab. If the object is on the bottom of the sclera (the white of the eye) or trapped under the lower lid, pull down on the lower lid and ask the patient to look up. If it is on the upper part of the sclera, pull up on the upper lid and ask the patient to look down. Wipe the object from the eye with the gauze or swab. If the object is trapped under the upper lid, pull the upper lid down over the lower lid, then release it. The lashes of the lower lid may sweep the object free. If that technique doesn't work, the upper lid can be carefully turned up and the object removed with a sterile gauze or sterile swab.

Field Treatment for Impaled Object

- When an object has become embedded in the eyeball, there should be no attempt to remove it in the field. Instead, the object should be stabilized in place if it extends beyond the surface of the face, or the eyeball may be covered with an eye shield.
- Do not apply ice packs to any injury to the globe.
- Arrange immediate transport to a trauma center.

Field Treatment for Laceration

- Apply eye shields to both eyes.
- Do not apply ice packs to any injury to the globe.
- Arrange immediate transport to a trauma center.

Chemical Burn

Chemical burns to the eye constitute a significant emergency, and time will be of the essence. If you are immediately aware of the mechanism of injury (that is, if you or others, including the patient, were a witness to the chemical being splashed or sprayed into the patient's eyes), you must begin treatment immediately. If the incident was not witnessed and the patient cannot provide any information, you must quickly evaluate the signs and symptoms to determine if a chemical burn has occurred. Signs and symptoms of a chemical burn include:

- Extreme pain in the eyes and the surrounding area
- Extreme redness in the eye
- Burned, inflamed, swollen or irritated skin surrounding the eye

Field Treatment for a Chemical Burn

- The only field treatment for a chemical burn is immediate and continuous flushing with clean water. The eyes should be flushed for at least 20 minutes (60 minutes for an alkali chemical burn) or until EMS reaches the patient or the patient reaches EMS. The eyes should be flushed from the inside out. In other words, the water should run from the eye to the side of the face, not from one eye to the other, which can cross-contaminate the eyes.
- Arrange immediate transport to a trauma center.

Applying an Eye Shield

For injuries to the globe, including penetrations and lacerations, an eye shield should be applied to protect the eye from further injury. Eye shields are available in aluminum or polycarbonate and should be applied using the technique on the opposite page.

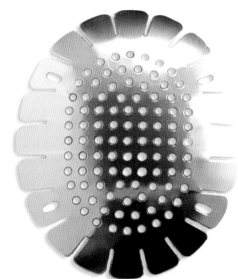

Fox Eye Shield
The Fox Eye Shield is available either in its basic configuration or with a soft cotton garter surrounding the outer perimeter of the shield.

To hear more about an innovative eye shield from H&H called the "Combat Eye Shield," see the "Additional Gear and Gadgets" section in Chapter 4.

Step 1: Place an aluminum or polycarbonate eye shield over the injured eye.

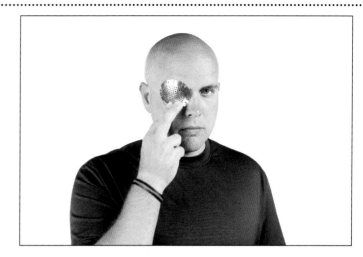

Step 2: Hold in place with rolled gauze, such as H&H Compressed Gauze.

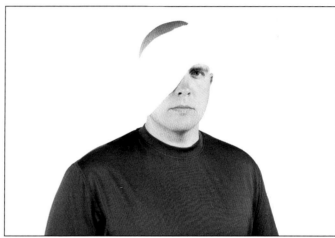

Step 3: Secure gauze in place with self-sticking tape, such as Coban or CoFlex.

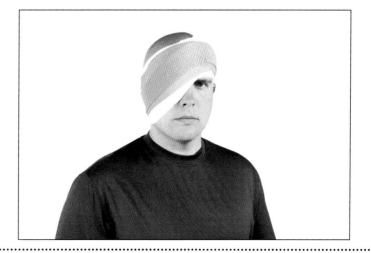

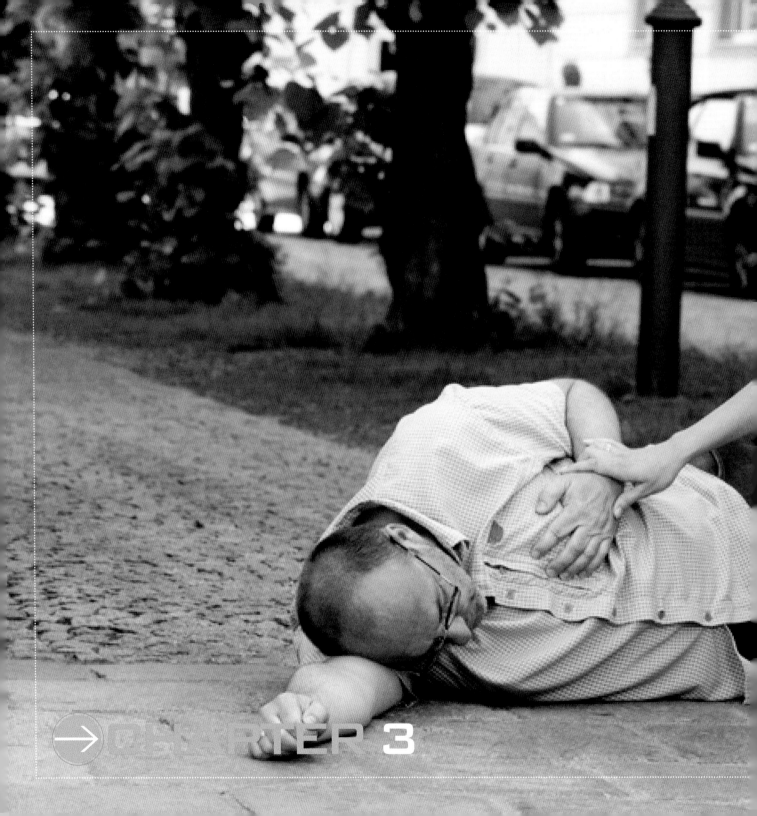

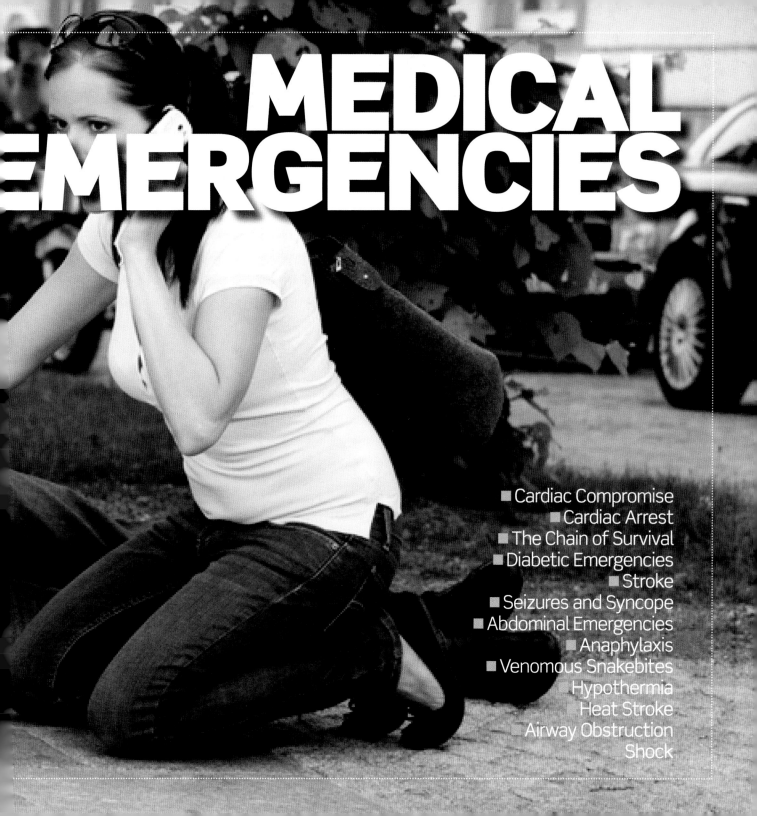

MEDICAL EMERGENCIES

- Cardiac Compromise
- Cardiac Arrest
- The Chain of Survival
- Diabetic Emergencies
- Stroke
- Seizures and Syncope
- Abdominal Emergencies
- Anaphylaxis
- Venomous Snakebites
- Hypothermia
- Heat Stroke
- Airway Obstruction
- Shock

magine you and your friends are preparing to embark on a hunting trip or a visit to the local gun range. What do you think would be the most likely emergency you would face? If you said, "A gunshot wound," it might surprise you to find out that in the United States, you are 1,110 times more likely to find yourself dealing with a stroke; 500 times more likely to deal with a cardiac arrest; and tens of thousands of times more likely to find yourself dealing with a diabetic emergency than you are to encounter a gunshot injury. While you should also know how to deal with a gunshot injury (which we addressed in Chapter 2), this chapter will deal with the medical emergencies mentioned above, — and several others.

Many of the medical emergencies that we'll discuss will require immediate action from bystanders if the patient is to stand a chance of surviving. That is especially true for the first medical emergency we'll discuss — cardiac arrest. That same immediate action is required for other emergencies outlined in this chapter including a severe allergic reaction referred to as anaphylaxis, severe environmental emergencies including hypothermia and heat stroke, severe abdominal emergencies, shock, and for cases when a patient is choking. Other medical emergencies have little or no field treatment that will change the outcome; instead, recognizing the condition will help the patient receive the proper interventions in an emergency room. Those conditions include stroke and a myocardial infarction (better known as a heart attack, which is different from cardiac arrest). Because of the importance of recognition in those cases, we'll dive a bit deeper than normal and explain the underlying causes of those medical conditions and their specific signs and symptoms. Lastly, we'll also discuss a number of medical emergencies which may or may not require transport to a hospital, but which still require a good assessment and good patient care. Those emergencies include diabetic emergencies and syncope (which is a fancy way of saying that the patient fainted).

While field treating the traumatic emergencies discussed in Chapter 2 often require specific gear or gadgets (such as tourniquets, compression bandages, SAM splints or a field expedient traction splint), the vast majority of the medical emergencies that will be reviewed in this chapter require nothing more than a pair of nitrile gloves, some critical thinking and someone to take a leadership role.

That person can be you.

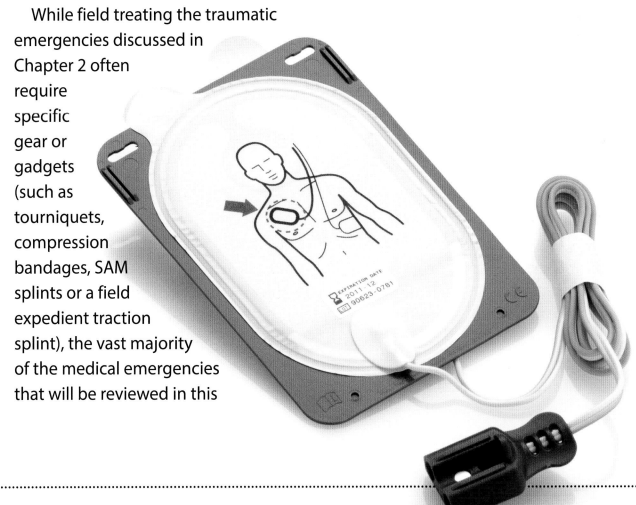

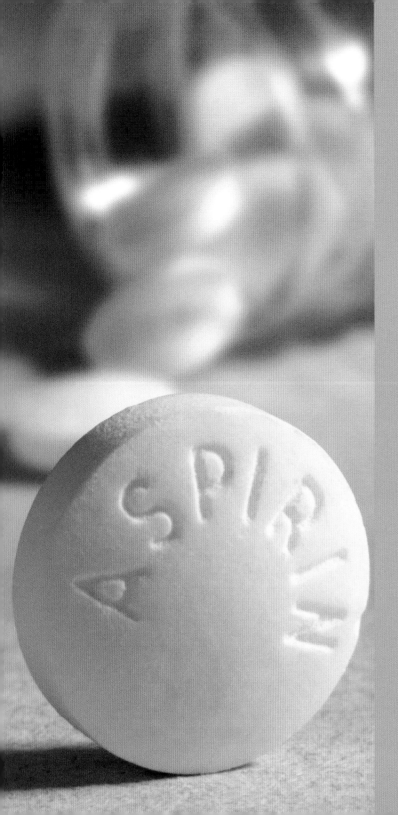

ASPIRIN
THE (ALMOST) WONDER DRUG

It's long been known that aspirin provides benefits far beyond easing the occasional headache or body ache. Through its antiplatelet properties (meaning, it prevents blood cells called platelets from clumping together and forming clots), aspirin has become a daily medication for millions of Americans who are at risk of heart attack or stoke (Never self-diagnose, or self-medicate — get advice from your doctor before making any medication decision). In the world of EMS, a bottle of baby aspirin typically sits in the "med" kit, next to more advanced drugs like morphine. Aspirin is well-known for increasing positives outcome for heart attack patients. In fact, many EMS protocols recommend 324 mg of aspirin (one adult aspirin, or four chewable children's aspirin) for patients exhibiting the symptoms of a heart attack — even prior to establishing whether a heart attack is actually occurring. So if you find yourself hours from EMS care and you or a loved one exhibits the symptoms discussed on the following page, even Harvard Medical School recommends popping four baby aspirin and getting to EMS care as quickly as possible. As with all medications, aspirin should only be taken by those who are not allergic to it. If you're unsure, consult your doctor.

CARDIAC COMPROMISE

Right behind traumatic injury, heart attack ranks as the second most-feared medical emergency while away from EMS coverage. Millions of Americans fear the telltale signs of a loved one suddenly clutching his or her chest in pain. They pray that if that day ever comes, EMS support and the emergency room will only be minutes away. While a heart attack might be the best-known of all cardiac compromises, there are a variety of reasons why someone's heart may stop beating. Those reasons might include drowning or suffocation; electrocution or lightning strike; or other medical reasons beyond a heart attack (or, a myocardial infarction, as it's better known in the EMS world). Severe asthma attacks or allergic reactions could also trigger an MI.

The methods to restart a heart are the same regardless of whether it was stopped by a heart attack or any other reason, but I'm going to begin this section by explaining a bit more about what exactly a heart attack entails.

Understanding Heart Attacks

Commonly referred to as a heart attack, a myocardial infarction results from a lack of oxygenated blood to the heart (that's right, the heart itself has its own set of blood vessels.) This may be a result of plaque buildup in those vessels or other causes. The lack of oxygenated blood will eventually lead to atrophy of a section of the heart muscle, which can cause a disruption in the electrical signals that travel through the heart. Like a complex piece of electronics, the heart muscle will only operate properly when those signals are sent and received in the proper order and when following the proper electrical paths. Any interruption to those signals can result in an MI.

Signs and Symptoms

While often characterized by chest pain, MIs can also be signaled by pain in the shoulder, arm or jaw. They can even occur as "silent MIs" which often occur in the elderly and in diabetics. Women in particular can have atypical MI symptoms, which is why you should see your doctor whenever you experience any symptoms out of the ordinary, such as those I've listed, or other symptoms such as unexplained fainting, the rapid onset of fatigue, unexplained shortness of breath or profuse sweating. If you suddenly experienced experienced massive chest pressure and pain radiating down your arm, you might automatically think, "I'm having a heart attack!" The reality is that most heart attack symptoms aren't so obvious and could be mistaken for fatigue, gas pains, or an everyday backache.

Field Treatment

- If you or another person presents with symptoms of an MI, call 911 immediately. This is not the type of medical condition that can wait, and it's not the type of condition that can be diagnosed or treated at your local clinic.
- If you find yourself hours from EMS care while you or a loved one exhibits such symptoms, Harvard Medical School recommends popping four baby aspirin and getting to EMS care as quickly as possible.

No doubt, an MI can be frightening. But there are now a number of life-saving treatments that can extend the life of the patient if caught in time. These include medications and surgical interventions. Ignore the signs and symptoms, and you might find yourself or a loved one moving from a cardia compromise to cardiac arrest.

A Heart Attack Waiting to Happen
Millions of Americans are one cheeseburger away from a heart attack as their coronary arteries become clogged with plaque. As the diameter of these arteries diminishes, the flow of oxygenated blood becomes less and less. The muscles of the heart begin to atrophy and die. Don't ignore the signs and symptoms of an MI.

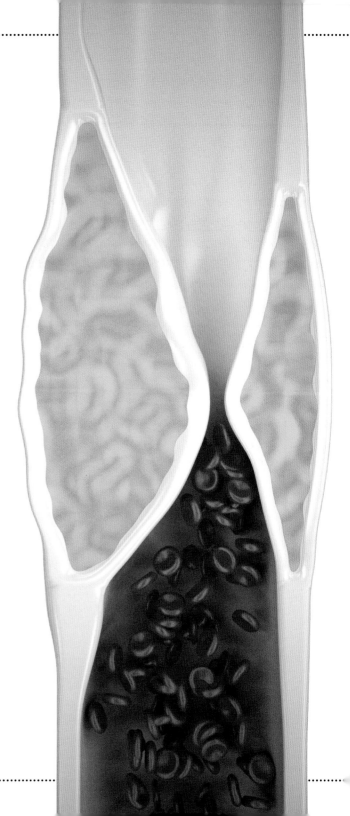

CARDIAC ARREST

The American Heart Association has developed what they refer to as the **Chain of Survival** when it comes to the survivability of a patient whose heart has stopped beating. The more quickly this condition can be recognized, the better. For this reason, it is imperative to immediately initiate the assessment that we covered in Chapter 1 upon identifying a traumatic or medical emergency. Within seconds, rescuers should be able to identify that the patient does not have a heartbeat, and the chain can be activated. On the next few pages, we'll follow the "Lay Rescuers" path shown below. I'll walk you through what your responsibilities will be at each step of the chain. I'll also briefly discuss what you should do when the ambulance arrives, which is link number four shown below.

1. Early Recognition

To recognize cardiac arrest, you should assess the patient for important signs and symptoms.

Signs and Symptoms

- Patient is unresponsive to verbal or painful stimulus.
- Patient is not breathing or is only gasping.
- Rescuers detect no carotid pulse after checking for 10 seconds.

2. Early Compressions

Upon recognizing cardiac arrest, you should call 911 and begin chest compressions — ideally within two minutes. American Heart Association studies have determined that during the first few minutes of a heart stopping, the blood will contain enough residual oxygen such that compressions alone can keep the brain oxygenated for several minutes. This is normally enough time to complete the remainder of the "Chain of Survival." The American Heart Association has found that compressions are *so* important that they've reordered the ABCs when dealing with cardiac emergencies, to CAB — Compressions, Airway and Breathing. Studies have shown that rescuers sometimes wasted precious

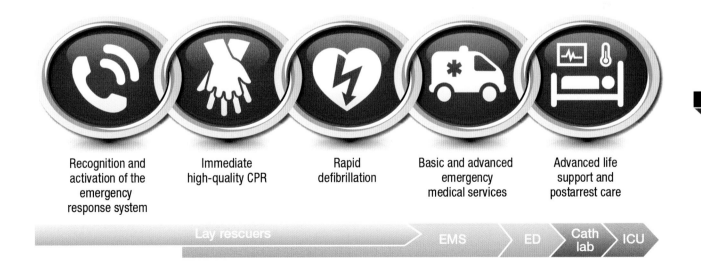

| Recognition and activation of the emergency response system | Immediate high-quality CPR | Rapid defibrillation | Basic and advanced emergency medical services | Advanced life support and postarrest care |

Lay rescuers   EMS   ED   Cath lab   ICU

minutes trying to open a patient's airway or begin rescue breaths. Those precious minutes should have been spent delivering fast and deep compressions.

Regardless of whether you are performing traditional CPR or "hands-only" CPR, the American Heart Association continues to recommend that you perform compressions at a rate of approximately **100 per minute**. If performing compressions and breaths, they should be done at a ratio of **30:2**. That is, 30 compressions, then two breaths (ideally, performed by a second rescuer). As funny as it might sound, an effective way to know that you're performing 100 compressions per minute is to hum a song in your head with the appropriate beat. The one recommended by the American Heart Association is "Stayin' Alive" by the Bee Gees, which is also very appropriate for the circumstances. (The song "Another One Bites the Dust" by Queen also works, but if the victim's family overhears you humming that one, they might be less appreciative of your efforts.)

The vast majority of individuals performing CPR on patients do not make the compressions nearly deep enough. EMS providers are often told that if they are providing deep enough compressions, they'll very often hear the ribs popping or cracking. While that may sound like you're doing more damage than good, you need to consider the alternative — in other words, your patient is already dead. While proper compressions may crack a rib, improper compressions will ensure that they remain dead.

When performing compressions, it is critical to have more than one rescuer share the task of delivering compressions. To properly compress an adult's chest to the proper depth of **two inches**, you must apply 100 - 125 pounds of pressure. That means that if you are performing CPR for even two minutes, it will be the equivalent of lifting 125 pounds, 2 inches, 200 times. That effort will exhaust even the strongest rescuer in just minutes.

The Clock is Ticking...

If you do not start CPR or defibrillation within 4 to 5 minutes of cardiac arrest, the heart will shift from the "electrical phase" to the "circulatory phase." During this time the body's oxygen and glucose reserves will have been exhausted and the heart will not be prepared for defibrillation. As a result, if a patient has been in cardiac arrest for longer than 4 to 5 minutes before you start CPR or defibrillation, you must perform two minutes of CPR before the use of an AED. If you haven't started resuscitation until ten minutes or more after cardiac arrest, the heart will be starved of oxygen and glucose and the patient's chances of survival will have dropped dramatically.

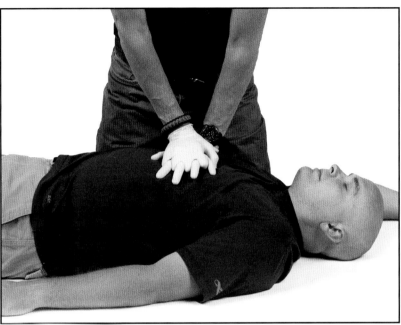

1 **Step 1:** After confirming that your patient is in cardiac arrest, have a bystander call 911 and another bystander find the closest AED.

2 **Step 2:** With your arms straight and your center of gravity over your hands, begin giving hard and deep compressions. The motion of your body should be in your hips, not in your arms (otherwise you'll be delivering completely ineffective "Hollywood" compressions). On an adult, your compressions should be approximately 2 inches deep. Deliver compressions at a rate of 100 per minute, at the same rate as the beat in the song, "Stayin' Alive" by the Bee Gees.

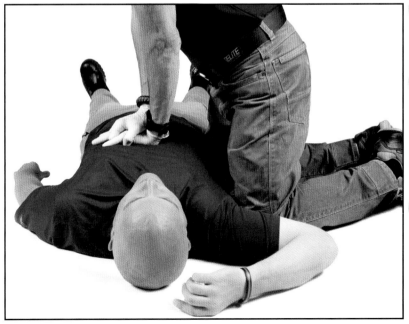

3 **Step 3:** Allow the chest to fully recoil between compressions.

4 **Step 4:** "Hands only" CPR can sustain the life of the patient if EMS arrives within minutes, but if help is farther out than that, you must also deliver rescue breaths. The compression to breath ratio should be 30:2, or 30 compressions then two breaths — ideally performed by two separate rescuers.

5 **Step 5:** Delivering compressions correctly can exhaust a rescuer in as few as 3 - 4 minutes. Rescuers should rotate tasks whenever one rescuer is becoming exhausted. **When rotating tasks, coordinate the rotation so that compressions are interrupted for no more than 10 seconds.**

3. Early Defibrillation

Since the popular series *Emergency!* premiered in 1972, television audiences have seen thousands of instances where medical professionals brought their patients back to life after rubbing conductive gel onto paddles, placing those paddles on their patient's chest, and shouting "clear!" What hasn't made its way onto

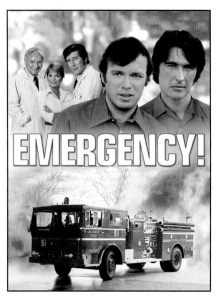

Emergency!
Running from 1972 to 1977, the TV show *Emergency!* spanned 129 episodes and 6 made-for-TV movies. Starring Randolph Mantooth and Kevin Tighe as Johnny Gage and Roy DeSoto, the show followed the two young firefighters as they progressed through the newly formed paramedic program at the fictional Fire Station 51 of the Los Angles Fire Department.

the air is that automatic external defibrillators (AEDs) are now so simple that even untrained individuals can follow the AED's simple, step-by-step robotic commands. Simply turning a modern AED on begins the process of verbal commands, such as, "Plug in leads," and "Place pads on patient's chest." As with all immediate life threats, timing is everything. Survival rates of patients who have "shockable rhythms" are as high as 49 to 75 percent if defibrillation is provided within the first 3 to 5 minutes after cardiac arrest. According to the American Heart Association, for every minute after that, the likelihood of survival drops by 7 to 10 percent.

For AEDs to work, they need to detect a "shockable rhythm," which would include ventricular tachycardia and ventricular fibrillation. In both of these rhythms, the electrical signals to the heart are disorganized and aren't providing appropriate signals for a proper heartbeat. When these electrical signals are completely absent, the heart is said to be in asystole. At that point, even an AED cannot resuscitate the patient. That means that if you and other rescuers debate for three or four minutes

ASYSTOLE
[ah-**sis**-toe-lee]
The absence of any electrical signals in the heart; flatline.

about what to do, you've most likely eliminated the chances that your patient can be revived. While AED models and procedures vary, most are now computer-operated and provide verbal instructions from the moment that you open the lid. For an example, see the step-by-step instructions on the following two pages.

Do you want to save a life? Look for this symbol wherever you go — at church, the grocery store, the library, the airport or your children's school. Know where to find the AED. In the event of a cardiac arrest, you'll know the location of this life-saving device. While you deliver hard and deep compressions, send a runner to quickly retrieve the AED.

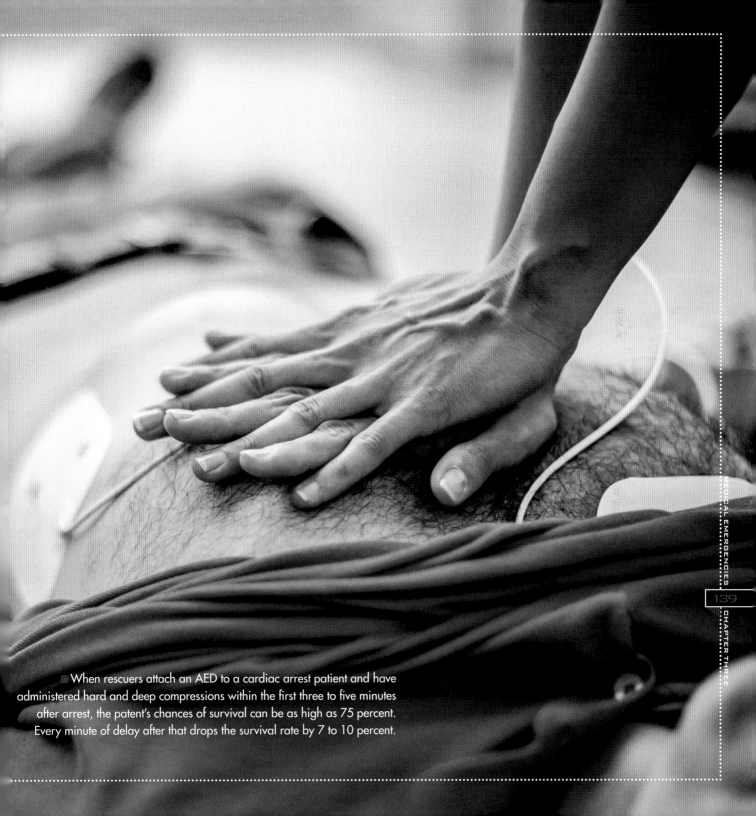

When rescuers attach an AED to a cardiac arrest patient and have administered hard and deep compressions within the first three to five minutes after arrest, the patent's chances of survival can be as high as 75 percent. Every minute of delay after that drops the survival rate by 7 to 10 percent.

1 Step 1: If the cardiac arrest occurred less than two minutes ago and the AED is immediately available, have one rescuer begin compressions while another rescuer begins deploying the AED. If the cardiac arrest was not witnessed, or if the down time is greater than four minutes, you should perform two minutes of CPR before attaching the AED.

2 Step 2: Although functionality varies between models, most AEDs go into automatic mode when either the lid is opened or the "On" button is pressed. This starts the voice prompts which will walk you through the rest of the process.

3 Step 3: The first command from the AED is typically to "Place pads on patient's chest." There are two pads; each will have a graphical representation of where it should be placed, as shown on the example on this page. Do NOT interrupt chest compressions for more than ten seconds while placing the chest pads. To work correctly, the pads must have a good connection on relatively dry skin, so if the patient's chest is wet or sweaty, wipe it with a shirt or towel before placing the pads.

If the person is wearing a medication patch that's in the same location that the pad should go, remove it and wipe any residual medicine from the skin before applying the pads.

Remove metal necklaces and underwire bras before applying the pads as the metal may conduct electricity and cause burns.

Lastly, check the patient for implanted medical devices, such as a pacemaker or implantable cardioverter defibrillator (the outline of these devices will be visible as a lump under the skin on the chest). Place the pads at least one inch away from these devices, even if that means they are not placed in the exact spot as in the graphic.

If the AED is not detecting a good connection, it will prompt you with a voice command such as, "Check pads." If the person has a lot of chest hair, it can interfere with the connection, and you may have to trim the hair before placing the pads. (Most AEDs will include a kit that contains a razor.) A method used by EMS to quickly remove chest hair is to attach one set of pads to the appropriate spot, and then rip them off quickly; think of this as a field-expedient method of waxing. Discard the first set of pads and apply the second set to the now-hairless spots. Believe me, if your patient is in cardiac arrest, they won't feel a thing.

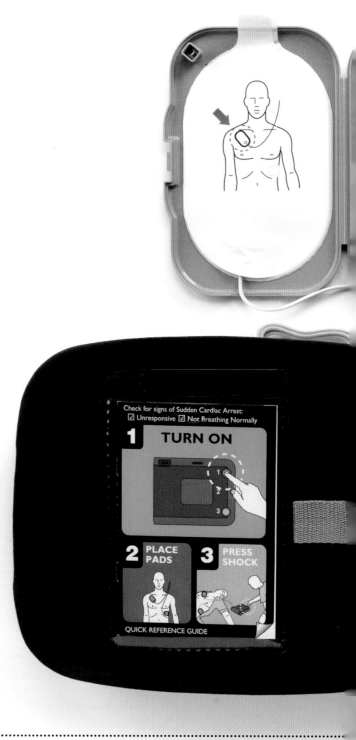

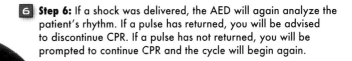

Step 4: If the pads are not already plugged into the AED, you will be directed to do so by the voice prompts. You may then be prompted to press an "Analyze" button, although most modern AEDs will automatically go into this mode with a voice prompt such as, "Analyzing patient. Stop CPR." At this point, you should stop CPR and stop touching the patient. Do not allow anyone to touch or bump the patient while the rhythm is being analyzed.

Step 5: After a short wait, the AED will advise you of the next step, either to shock the patient or to continue CPR. If you are advised to begin CPR, it is because the AED did not detect a shockable rhythm. If it advises you to shock the patient, it will make a voice prompt such as, "Shock advised. Stand clear of the patient, and press the shock button." At this point, you and other rescuers should ensure that no part of your body is touching the patient. The rescuer in charge of the AED should confirm this by saying, "Don't touch the patient." When everyone is confirmed clear, you should say, "Shocking" and press the "Shock" button.

Step 6: If a shock was delivered, the AED will again analyze the patient's rhythm. If a pulse has returned, you will be advised to discontinue CPR. If a pulse has not returned, you will be prompted to continue CPR and the cycle will begin again.

4. Early Advanced Life Services

Advanced life service providers (known as ALS, or paramedics who would arrive on the ambulance) can provide life-sustaining drugs and other interventions, increasing the likelihood of a positive outcome for your patient. The faster you can get the ambulance to your patient, the better. With everything else you have going on, don't forget that call to 911 at the start of the chain.

When the Ambulance Arrives

When the ambulance arrives on the scene, you should continue with compressions and wait for the ambulance crew's instructions. They will want to know:

- What the "down time" was (when the cardiac arrest occurred).
- When CPR was started.
- If any shocks were delivered.
- If any family members or friends are present, the crew will also want to know if the patient has any pertinent history that they should know about, and what preceded the cardiac arrest. For example, they'll want to know if something other than an MI caused the arrest, such as electrocution or an allergic reaction.

If the ambulance crew believes that you are providing adequate compressions, they may ask you to continue doing so while they prepare their life-saving gear. This may include a LUCAS device designed to deliver mechanical compressions powered by a battery or compressed air. They will prepare one or more IVs or IOs (intraosseous infusion, which is a process of drilling a hole directly into the marrow of a bone to provide an entry point for fluids and medication) and they will prepare a number of medications designed to restart your patient's heart. Such medications may include epinephrine, amiodarone and vasopressin. They may also remove the AED pads that are attached to the patient and attach their own pads, which will deliver shocks from their monitor. Unlike an AED, the paramedic's monitor can adjust the power (measured in joules) of the shocks delivered. For example, they may make a weight-based calculation for a child, which would lower the strength of the shock when compared with an adult.

One fact that many bystanders find surprising after the ambulance arrives at the scene of a cardiac arrest is that the EMTs and paramedics will continue to work on the patient at the scene of the cardiac arrest (sometimes for an hour or more), rather than immediately loading the patient on the ambulance and transporting them to an emergency room. The reality is, when it comes to cardiac arrest, the care provided by an ALS crew on the scene will be no different than the care provided at the emergency room. Disrupting chest compressions, medications, and the delivery of shocks to load a patient on the ambulance may have a detrimental effect. As a result, most ALS crews will continue to work a cardiac arrest patient on the scene until the patient either has a return of spontaneous circulation (ROSC), or until the lead paramedic or medical control officially calls it.

HOW IMPORTANT IS THAT CALL TO 911?
MANY PATIENT OUTCOMES ARE MEASURED IN MINUTES

So just how important is that phone call to 911? In the case of cardiac arrest, stroke or serious trauma, the patient's outcome is often measured in minutes. For example, the American Heart Association has determined that three phases occur during cardiac arrest — the electrical phase, which lasts from 0 minutes (the moment the arrest occurs) to 4 minutes; the circulatory phase which lasts from 4 to 10 minutes; and the metabolic phase, which begins 10 minutes after the arrest.

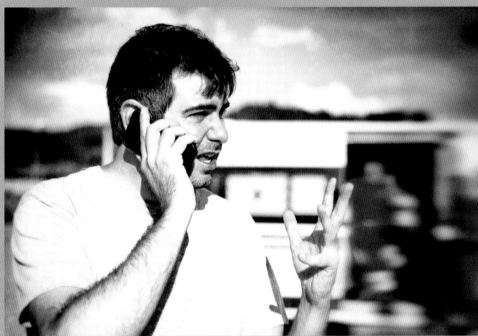

During the electrical phase, the heart and bloodstream still have a good supply of oxygen and glucose, and even "hands only" CPR will continue to circulate that oxygen and glucose. During this phase, the heart is ready for immediate defibrillation. If rescuers do not initiate CPR or defibrillation during this phase, the heart will have shifted into the circulatory phase. During this second stage, the body's oxygen and glucose reserves have been exhausted and the heart will not be prepared for defibrillation. Because of this, if a patient has been in cardiac arrest for longer than 4 minutes before the start of CPR or defibrillation, it will be necessary to perform 2 minutes of CPR before the use of an AED. If resuscitation hasn't been started until 10 minutes or more after the cardiac arrest, the heart will be starved of oxygen and glucose, and the patient's chances of survival will have dropped dramatically. Similarly, patients who have experienced an ischemic stroke (a stroke caused by a blocked vessel in the brain) must be transported to an emergency room within 2 hours of the stroke so they can receive a fibrinolytic drug within a 3-hour window. After that 3-hour window closes, the likelihood of a positive outcome drops by 33 percent.

UNDERSTANDING DIABETES

According to the CDC, more than 25 million Americans suffer from either Type 1 or Type 2 diabetes. Even with that large percentage of the population being directly affected by the disease, many people incorrectly believe that diabetes is a disease of *low* blood sugar. In fact it's the opposite. The disease can cause dramatically elevated levels of blood sugar (or blood glucose as it's more appropriately called) if left untreated. In what will sound like a direct contradiction to that statement, most diabetic emergencies occur because a patient's blood glucose has dropped to dangerously low levels. To understand that contradiction, let me explain a bit about insulin and glucose and why the body — most importantly the brain — requires a careful balance of those two important molecules. Glucose is a major source of energy for our body's cells, including our brain cells. But, in order for glucose to move into those cells, insulin, which is produced by the pancreas, must first attach itself to the cell. Insulin effectively acts as a "key" to allow glucose to pass through the cell membrane.

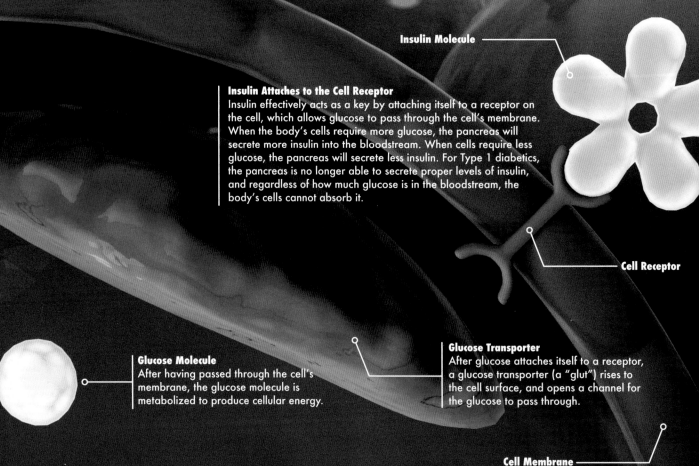

Insulin Molecule

Insulin Attaches to the Cell Receptor
Insulin effectively acts as a key by attaching itself to a receptor on the cell, which allows glucose to pass through the cell's membrane. When the body's cells require more glucose, the pancreas will secrete more insulin into the bloodstream. When cells require less glucose, the pancreas will secrete less insulin. For Type 1 diabetics, the pancreas is no longer able to secrete proper levels of insulin, and regardless of how much glucose is in the bloodstream, the body's cells cannot absorb it.

Cell Receptor

Glucose Molecule
After having passed through the cell's membrane, the glucose molecule is metabolized to produce cellular energy.

Glucose Transporter
After glucose attaches itself to a receptor, a glucose transporter (a "glut") rises to the cell surface, and opens a channel for the glucose to pass through.

Cell Membrane

The common form of diabetes, *diabetes mellitus*, results from a lack of insulin being secreted by the pancreas, resulting in dramatically elevated blood glucose levels, or what's referred to as **hyperglycemia** ("hyper" means "high"). Type 1 diabetes, also referred to as "Insulin Dependent Diabetes," requires the patient to inject or inhale insulin to replace the insulin normally produced by the pancreas. When a diabetic emergency occurs, the culprit is usually not the underlying disease itself. Instead, It's usually because something has gone wrong with the management of the disease. For example, it may occur because the patient has taken too much insulin; or they've taken their normal amount of insulin but have skipped a meal; or, it can be caused if they exert themselves more than normal, which burns more glucose than usual. In all of those cases, the careful balance of insulin and glucose is thrown out of whack, and the proper amount of glucose in the blood drops below a safe level. In fact, most people will be in an altered mental state when their blood glucose drops below 60 mg/dL (the normal range is 80—120 mg/dL). This state is often mistaken for intoxication. If the diabetic patient recognizes the signs and symptoms of low blood sugar, they're usually able to solve the problem by eating a high-sugar food, drinking fruit juice or ingesting

something similar. If you are on a camping, hiking or canoe trip with an individual who has Type 1 diabetes, you must also be able to recognize the signs and symptoms of low blood sugar, or **hypoglycemia** ("hypo" means "low") as explained below.

Signs and Symptoms

- An altered mental status, which may present itself as intoxication
- Moist, cool skin
- An elevated heart rate
- Anxiousness, restlessness, or uncharacteristic combativeness

Field Treatment

If these signs and symptoms present themselves, you should ask the patient if they are a diabetic, or check their wrist for a medical bracelet. Treatment can usually be accomplished by asking the patient if they are able to eat a small amount of high-sugar food or drink a high-sugar fluid. If the patient is unable to do that or is completely unresponsive, you must get your patient to EMS, or EMS to your patient, as soon as possible.

UNDERSTANDING STROKE

After cardiac arrest, stroke is the most-feared medical condition for most adults past their 50s and 60s — with good cause. According to the American Heart Association, stroke is the third leading cause of death, with more than 700,000 people suffering a stroke each year. Upwards of 160,000 of those patients die as a consequence.

So what exactly is a stroke? Recall the underlying causes of a heart attack, where a portion of the heart muscle receives an inadequate level of blood. Those same conditions are at play here, but in this case, the damage is occurring within the brain. In a heart attack, a coronary artery is being blocked. During a stroke, a cerebral artery is blocked by a clot or the artery has ruptured.

Early recognition of the stroke means early transport to an emergency room and early treatment. Drugs and mechanical devices can treat stroke patients, even reversing the consequences of the stroke, by breaking up the clot that caused the obstruction. But these drugs must be administered within 3 hours of the onset of the symptoms. To accomplish this, rescuers must deliver the patient to the emergency room within *two* hours of the onset.

To remember what to do if you believe someone is experiencing a stroke, we use the acronym FAST. The first three letters are reminders on how to identify stroke symptoms. Look for stroke symptoms in the patient's face, arms and ability to speak. A stroke may cause deficits in one or more of these areas. For example, if your patient shows an uneven smile, is experiencing weakness in one arm, or is slurring his or her speech, he or she may be experiencing a stroke. To test these three conditions, we use a simple test in the field called the **Cincinnati Pre-Hospital Stroke Scale**. First, ask your patient to give you a full-face smile. Look for any unevenness in the smile, such as drooping lips

FACE **AR**M **S**PEECH **T**IME

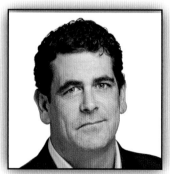

Does one side of the face droop or is it numb? Ask the person to smile.

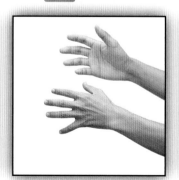

Is one arm weak or numb? Ask the person to raise both arms, palms up. Does one arm drift?

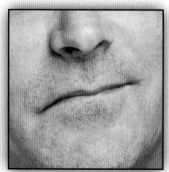

Is the speech slurred, are they unable to speak or difficult to understand? Ask them to repeat a simple sentence. Is the sentence repeated correctly?

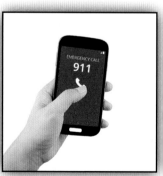

If the person shows any of these symptoms, even if the symptoms go away, call 911 and get them to the hospital immediately.

on one side of the patient's face. Next, ask the patient to close his or her eyes and extend both arms to the front, palms up. Stroke patients will very often show an immediate drift down or to the side with one arm. Third, ask your patient to repeat a very simple phrase. In my agency, we ask our patients to repeat the phrase, "You can't teach an old dog new tricks." If the patient is unable to repeat that phrase word for word, or slur some of the words, he or she may be experiencing a stroke.

So what does the "T" stand for in the word FAST? It stands for Time. It's a reminder that if you believe the potential patient is experiencing a stroke, you must immediately call 911 and get that patient to an emergency room as quickly as possible. I will stress that there is *no field treatment* for a stroke. Early recognition and early delivery to the emergency room are the only treatments.

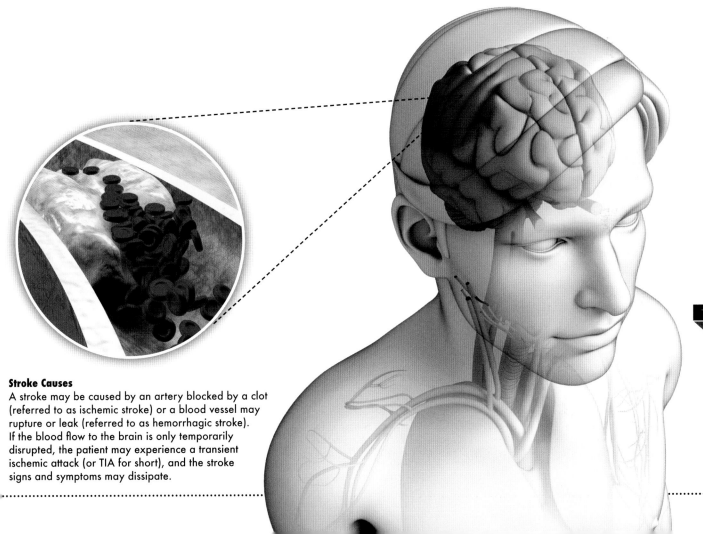

Stroke Causes
A stroke may be caused by an artery blocked by a clot (referred to as ischemic stroke) or a blood vessel may rupture or leak (referred to as hemorrhagic stroke). If the blood flow to the brain is only temporarily disrupted, the patient may experience a transient ischemic attack (or TIA for short), and the stroke signs and symptoms may dissipate.

SEIZURES

A seizure is a sudden and abnormal disruption of brain function caused by a massive electrical discharge affecting a portion of the brain and nervous system. Seizures are not considered a disease in and of themselves, but rather a symptom

An Electrical Storm in the Brain

Any disruption in the electrical signals of the brain can have a cascading effect throughout the rest of the nervous system. During a seizure, the brain is suddenly overwhelmed by a massive electrical discharge, which may lead to unconsciousness. If the disruption follows the nerve pathways (the yellow lines on the illustration to the right), it may result in a tonic-clonic (grand mal) seizure including muscle rigidity or uncontrolled muscle spasms.

of an underlying disease. Seizures could also result from an underlying medical condition such as a high fever or traumatic head injury.

Epilepsy

The most common disease related to seizure is epilepsy. An estimated 3 million Americans live with epilepsy today. Each year, doctors diagnose approximately 125,000 - 200,000 new cases. Epileptic seizures do not always occur as portrayed on television or in the movies. In fact, many seizures happen with no outward seizing activity. Instead, the patient may appear to be distracted, daydreaming or having some other minor behavioral disturbance.

However, during a grand mal seizure (more properly called a tonic-clonic seizure), the patient will progress through a number of phases, including:

Unconsciousness where the patient may momentarily lose consciousness.

The tonic phase where they will experience extreme muscle rigidity.

The clonic phase where the muscles will spasm repeatedly. During this phase, the diaphragm may also

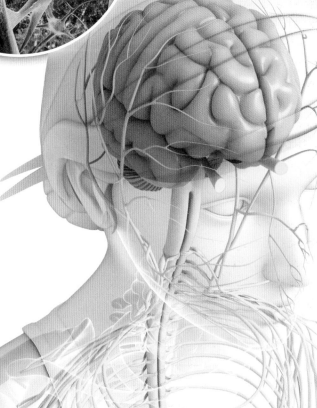

POSTICTAL
[pose-**tic**-tall]

A phase of recovery after a seizure where the patient may experience disorientation, confusion and weakness.

convulse, causing the patient to temporarily stop breathing or breathing may be extremely shallow.

The postictal phase is the end of the event. During the postictal phase, the patient may experience disorientation, confusion and weakness or may become combative. This phase may last 30 minutes or more. After the postictal phase, the patient may be fully alert and oriented, but may still be physically weak and need recovery time due to the massive muscle contractions. The postictal phase cannot be hurried — do not force your patient into answering questions, drinking any liquids or moving around until he or she is ready.

Other Causes

In addition to epilepsy and other underlying diseases, external factors including head trauma, hypoxia (a lack of oxygen to the brain), drug overdose, drug withdrawal, fever or infection can also induce seizures. Since seizures can have many causes, it's important not to get "tunnel vision" and make an incorrect assumption that your seizure patient has epilepsy. If you find yourself at the side of a patient in seizure or who is already postictal, you should attempt to make a determination about what might have caused the seizure. If the patient

SEIZURES
EMERGENCY CARE

Here's what you should do if you find yourself with a patient who has experienced a seizure:

- If the patient is still in seizure, simply protect him to ensure that he does not injure himself.
- After the patient emerges from seizure, assess his ABCs, and perform a rapid trauma assessment to determine if he injured himself during the seizure.
- Until you have confirmation that the patient has an underlying disease (such as epilepsy), be alert for traumatic or medical conditions, such as a head injury, that may have caused the seizure. Be aware that medical conditions such as heart attacks or stroke can be mistaken for seizures or may have caused the seizure. Don't assume that just because your patient is emerging from the postictal phase that he is out of danger.
- While the patient is postictal, continue to monitor his airway and breathing.
- As the patient emerges from the postictal phase, reassure him and let him know that EMS is on their way.
- Be aware that even after the postictal phase has ended, the patient may be so exhausted from the muscle contractions that they faint or fall asleep. This is particularly true for infants and toddlers.

is able to answer questions, he or she will be your best source of information. If they are not, you should perform a patient assessment, including a rapid trauma assessment, to ensure the patient's ABCs are adequate and that there is no underlying trauma that could have caused the seizure.

Febrile Seizure

Seizures involving infants or toddlers can be particularly terrifying. One common cause of seizure in young children is a spike in temperature, which can cause a type of seizure referred to as a febrile seizure.

> # FEBRILE SEIZURE
> [**feb**-rull]
> A seizure caused by a spike in temperature. Most common in children between 6 months and 5 years old.

Febrile seizures most typically occur in children between 6 months and 5 years old. As with all seizures, a febrile seizure requires immediate emergency medical care.

FAINTING (SYNCOPE)

Fainting, more properly called syncope, is often confused with a seizure because it may present with similar signs and symptoms including momentary unconsciousness and involuntary jerking of the muscles. Although seizures and syncope might present in a similar manner, their root causes and recoveries are very different. Instead of being triggered by massive electrical discharges in the brain, a syncopal episode has a simpler and better-understood explanation: a temporary lack of oxygen to the brain caused by a sudden drop in blood pressure. A common scenario just prior to a syncopal episode occurs when a patient has been sitting for a lengthy period of time, which allows blood to pool in the lower extremities. If the individual suddenly stands up, adequate blood flow to the brain may be temporarily interrupted as the cardiac system suddenly has to push blood several feet higher. Other syncopal episodes can be caused by the vagus nerve, which may unexpectedly dilate the vessels. This doesn't change the volume of blood, but it does change the volume of the vessels containing the blood. This could cause blood to suddenly pool around the lower extremities, diminishing the amount of blood perfusing the brain. When other factors are at play such as excessive heat or when the patient is already weakened due to low blood sugar or dehydration, the patient may be even more susceptible to an episode.

Most syncopal episodes occur when the patient is standing or has just stood up. The episode basically tells the patient to "get horizontal, now!" to allow adequate blood flow to return to the brain. If we were still prehistoric humans and the only danger was falling onto a soft rainforest floor, there would be little danger in a syncopal episode. In today's world, if a standing adult

> # SYNCOPE
> [**sink**-a-pee]
> A temporary loss of consciousness due to a lack of oxygen to the brain because of a sudden drop in blood pressure.

suddenly drops to the floor, they risk striking their head on a sharp object on the way down to a hard surface.

Not only is the root cause of syncopal episodes different than seizure, the recovery time is often quite different as well. Seizure patients often require 30 minutes or more of recovery time as they progress through the postictal phase of the seizure. By contrast, a patient who has experienced a syncopal episode will recover much faster, usually in minutes or almost immediately.

As with all medical conditions, it's important to perform a proper assessment to determine if something more serious is at play, such as a diabetic emergency, and to determine if the syncopal episode caused any trauma as the patient went from vertical to horizontal.

Field Treatment

- If the patient is still unconscious, monitor his or her airway.
- When the patient has recovered consciousness, keep them in a reclined position to allow adequate blood flow to the brain.
- If they the patient is in an environment that may have led to the syncopal episode (such as extreme heat), assist him or her out of the environment.
- Since most syncopal patients will recover quickly, he or she will be able to advise you on what, if any, further assistance you can provide.
- If the patient continues to have an altered mental status for more than a few minutes after the episode, you may consider that the episode was in fact a seizure. You should contact EMS immediately in this instance.

Because rescuers often confuse seizures with syncope, the table below offers a summary of the differences in cause, the signs and symptoms normally seen during the event, and the differences in recovery. If in doubt, assume your patient has had a seizure and respond accordingly.

SEIZURE	SYNCOPE
Root Cause	
Seizures are caused by massive electrical discharge in the brain.	The patient experiences a temporary loss of oxygen to the brain, usually caused by a sudden drop in blood pressure.
Signs and Symptoms During Event	
Seizures may present as distraction, daydreaming or some other minor behavioral disturbance. A tonic-clonic seizure will present with unconsciousness followed by extreme muscle rigidity, after which the muscles will spasm repeatedly.	The patient experiences a temporary loss of consciousness which may include involuntary jerking of the muscles.
Recovery Phase	
The postictal (recovery) phase may last up to 30 minutes or more. Patient may be disoriented, confused, weak or combative.	The patient will normally recover within minutes, particularly if they are placed in a seated or supine position which allows blood flow to return quickly to the brain.

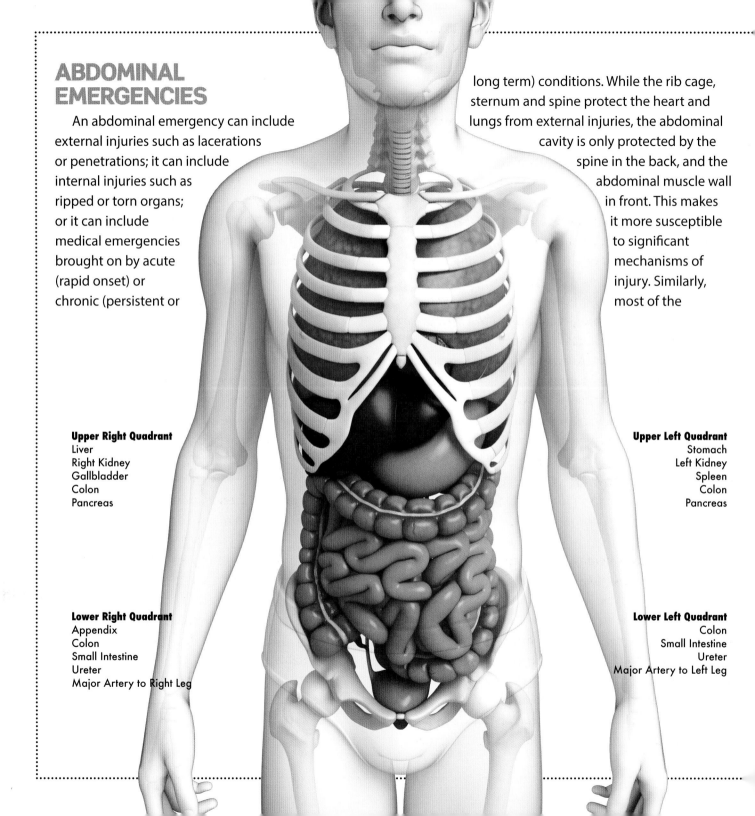

ABDOMINAL EMERGENCIES

An abdominal emergency can include external injuries such as lacerations or penetrations; it can include internal injuries such as ripped or torn organs; or it can include medical emergencies brought on by acute (rapid onset) or chronic (persistent or long term) conditions. While the rib cage, sternum and spine protect the heart and lungs from external injuries, the abdominal cavity is only protected by the spine in the back, and the abdominal muscle wall in front. This makes it more susceptible to significant mechanisms of injury. Similarly, most of the

Upper Right Quadrant
Liver
Right Kidney
Gallbladder
Colon
Pancreas

Upper Left Quadrant
Stomach
Left Kidney
Spleen
Colon
Pancreas

Lower Right Quadrant
Appendix
Colon
Small Intestine
Ureter
Major Artery to Right Leg

Lower Left Quadrant
Colon
Small Intestine
Ureter
Major Artery to Left Leg

abdominal organs are enclosed within a membrane called peritoneum while the pancreas, kidneys, uterus and abdominal aorta are located behind the peritoneum.

There are three general types of organs within the abdominal cavity: solid organs, hollow organs and vascular structures. Solid organs contain a large amount of blood and blood vessels that if ruptured or penetrated will result in internal bleeding, possibly leading to shock. Solid organs include the spleen, liver, pancreas and kidneys. Hollow organs do not contain a large number of blood vessels and will not bleed as much as solid organs if they are ruptured or penetrated. However, the substance within the hollow organ will leak into the abdominal cavity, which can irritate or inflame the lining of the peritoneum. Hollow organs include the stomach, gallbladder, duodenum, large intestine, small intestine and bladder. Vascular structures include the descending aorta and the inferior vena cava. Penetrations, ruptures or other injuries to these vessels will result in significant internal bleeding, shock and death.

Abdominal Pain

Abdominal pain can be divided into three categories: visceral pain, referred pain and parietal pain.

Visceral Pain

Visceral pain is pain radiating from the organ itself. However, since most abdominal organs do not contain a significant number of nerve endings (other than the liver, spleen and gallbladder), visceral pain will typically be felt as a dull ache which is difficult to localize. In other words, the patient may describe the pain as being dull,

intermittent and general in nature rather than being able to pinpoint an exact location.

Referred Pain

Referred pain is a variation of visceral pain and occurs when the organ shares nerve pathways with another part of the body. That shared nerve pathway will confuse the brain and may cause the patient to feel pain elsewhere on the body rather than localized near the organ itself. For example, a patient who has experienced an injury, rupture or inflammation of the gallbladder may actually feel the pain as a dull ache in the right shoulder blade.

Parietal Pain

Parietal pain occurs when blood or another substance leaking from an injured organ irritates or inflames the lining of the peritoneum — causing a condition referred to as peritonitis. The peritoneum contains a significant number of nerve endings. If irritated, it will cause pain that is more pronounced and localized, which will make it easier for the patient to articulate. The degree and onset of the pain will be dependent upon which organ or organs are leaking into the abdominal cavity. For example, the ileum (the third portion of the small intestine) contains digestive fluid with a neutral pH. If this fluid leaks into the peritoneum, pain may be dull, delayed or intermittent. On the other hand, the duodenum (the first part of the small intestine) contains a digestive substance that is highly acidic and would typically cause more localized, more intense and more immediate pain.

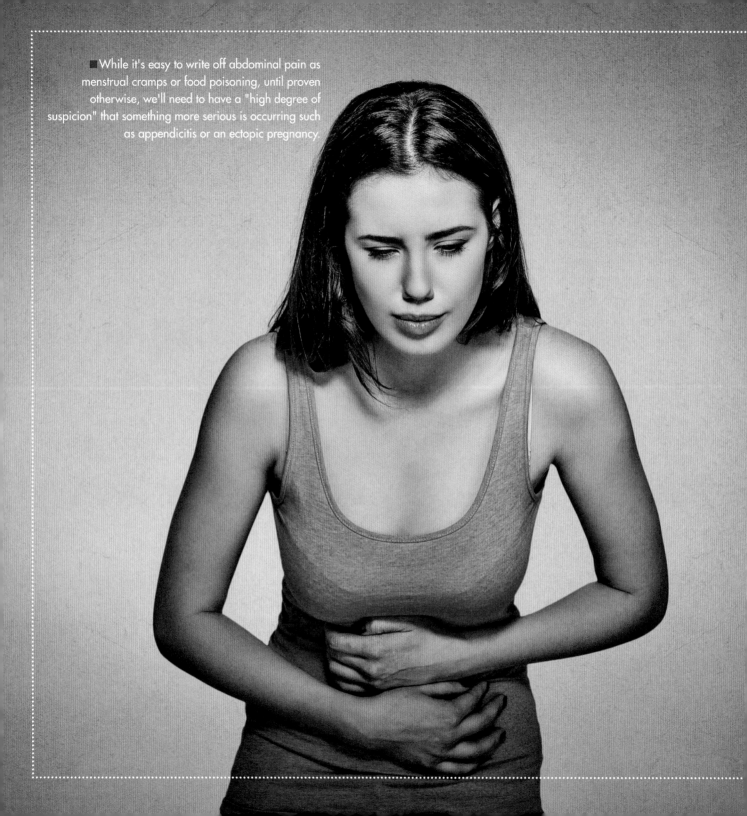

While it's easy to write off abdominal pain as menstrual cramps or food poisoning, until proven otherwise, we'll need to have a "high degree of suspicion" that something more serious is occurring such as appendicitis or an ectopic pregnancy.

A High Degree of Suspicion

Because of the myriad potential causes for abdominal pain and the fact that pain can be dull or severe, general, localized or referred — not to mention constant or intermittent — you should consider all abdominal pain to be serious until proven otherwise. As a nonprofessional rescuer, it's important that you not to fall into the trap of attempting to diagnose the underlying cause of abdominal pain. Instead, you must treat the signs and symptoms, including being prepared to treat the patient for shock, and to arrange for rapid transport to an emergency room.

In the EMS world, we use the phrase, "maintain a high degree of suspicion." What that means is that when we're presented with a set of signs and symptoms, we first evaluate the most significant reason that could be causing those signs and symptoms before concluding that the actual cause is something less serious. A common scenario used during EMT and paramedic training is to present a new trainee with a female patient who is complaining of lower abdominal pain. If the female was of childbearing age, a common assumption may be that the patient is simply experiencing pain from her menstrual cycle. Yet the goal of the scenario is to have the EMT or paramedic candidate evaluate what other, more serious medical conditions could be causing the pain, such as appendicitis or an ectopic pregnancy

(a very serious and life-threatening condition where a fertilized egg has become implanted in a fallopian tube rather than in the uterus). On the other hand, a "high degree of suspicion" doesn't mean that every ache and pain should be interpreted as a significant, life-threatening medical condition. It just mean that the most serious condition should be assumed until proven otherwise. In reality, that proof may need to occur in an emergency room rather than at your home or campsite.

The Markle "Heel Drop" Test

As mentioned, most patient assessment for abdominal pain is best left for the emergency room. That said, EMTs and paramedics do employ a field assessment technique which can add strength to the suspicion that the abdominal pain is being caused by either appendicitis or peritonitis. To perform the Markle test, the patient is asked to stand, then raise herself up onto her toes and then drop suddenly to cause an audible "thump." If the heel drop causes the patient to experience sharp, localized abdominal pain (or if you witness a grimace on your patient's face), it can add to your suspicion that the condition is something more serious than gas pain. If your patient is unable to stand, an alternate to the heel drop test can be performed by making a fist and striking the bottom of your patient's heel. This will jar your patient's torso similar to the standing heel drop test and should elicit the same response.

ECTOPIC PREGNANCY
[ek-**to**-pick]
A serious and life-threatening condition where a fertilized egg has become implanted in a fallopian tube rather than the uterus.

Appendicitis Signs and Symptoms

   Appendicitis is one of the most feared (and most imagined) medical conditions that can occur when outside of the umbrella of EMS. As such, I'll add some additional signs and symptoms here so you may adjust your "degree of suspicion" that you or another individual may be suffering from appendicitis. Signs and symptoms can include:

- Pain localized to the lower right quadrant, or dull pain centered around the navel
- Chills and a low-grade fever
- Abdominal guarding
- A positive Markle test

Field Treatment

   Regardless of whether an abdominal emergency is due to a medical condition or trauma, the following treatment should be performed:

- Monitor the patient's ABCs and prepare to treat for shock.
- Place the patient in a position of comfort, which will normally be in a reclined, or supine position. If the patient has experienced no injury to the lower extremities or the spine, the legs may be flexed at the

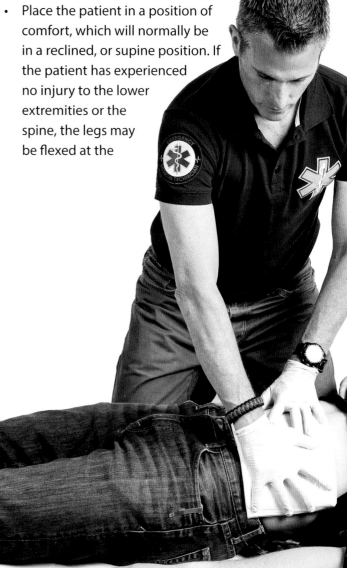

knees and positioned near the chest, which can reduce the pain experienced by the patient.
- Do not allow the patient to eat or drink anything.

Treatment for Evisceration

If the abdominal emergency is due to external trauma such as a laceration or penetration, you should expose the injury and perform this additional treatment:

- Cover the injury with a sterile dressing or a clean towel that has been soaked with sterile water. Place the dressing over any protruding organs (do not attempt to replace the organs back into the abdominal cavity). Cover the moist dressing with an occlusive dressing such as plastic wrap. This will retain the moisture on the dressing and keep the exposed organs from drying out.
- Seek immediate evacuation for the patient.

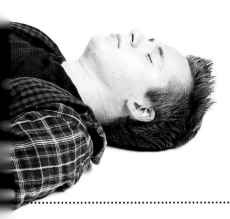

ABDOMINAL INJURIES
EMERGENCY CARE

Here's what you should do if you find yourself with a patient who has an abdominal emergency:

- Monitor the patient's ABCs, and prepare to treat for shock.
- Place the patient in a position of comfort, which will normally be in a reclined position (referred to as the supine position). If the patient has not sustained an injury to the lower extremities or the spine, the legs may be flexed at the knees and positioned near the chest, which can reduce pain.
- Do not allow the patient to eat or drink anything.

Additional Treatment for an Evisceration:

- Cover the injury with a sterile dressing or a clean towel that has been soaked with sterile water. Place the dressing over any protruding organs but do not attempt to replace the organs back into the abdominal cavity. Cover the moist dressing with an occlusive dressing such as plastic wrap.
- Seek immediate evacuation for the patient.

ANAPHYLAXIS

Millions of Americans suffer through seasonal or other non-life threatening allergies. But an anaphylactic reaction is an extreme, systematic, life-threatening allergic reaction that inflicts significant swelling of the upper and lower airways, constriction of the bronchioles, leakage of fluid from the capillaries and systematic blood vessel dilation (referred to as vasodilation). Common causes of anaphylactic reactions include food such as peanuts, shellfish, milk or eggs; venom from insect stings, such as those from bees or wasps; or certain medications, such as penicillin. If the patient has a known allergy, there is a very good chance they will already have a prescribed epinephrine auto-injector, often referred to as an "EpiPen."

Signs and Symptoms
- Patient has come into contact with their known allergen.
- Flushed skin, warm to the touch, caused by the dilation of the blood vessels.
- Swelling of the skin, lips, tongue, hands and feet, caused by the capillaries leaking into the epidermis (the outer layer of the skin).
- The presence of hives (raised red blotches) on the skin, accompanied by intense itching.
- A rapid and weak pulse. Decreased blood pressure, resultant of the dilated blood vessels, may render the radial pulse absent.
- Wheezing or crowing when the patient breathes, caused by a swollen upper airway.

Field Treatment
If the patient has an auto-injector, that must be the primary and immediate intervention whenever the patient has come into contact with their known allergen. Treatments such as Benadryl may relieve some early symptoms such as hives, but those early symptoms serve as warning signs that the patient is experiencing an anaphylactic reaction. Masking those early symptoms may delay critical epinephrine until it is too late.

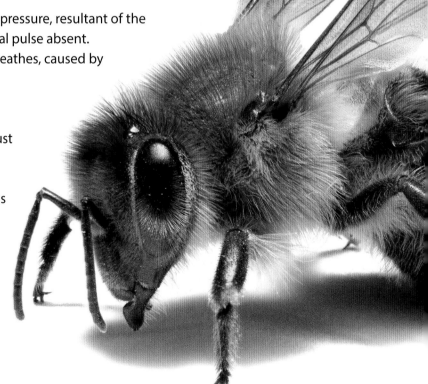

STINGING INSECTS

No one wants to be stung by a bee, but for an estimated 2 to 3 percent of the population, bee stings may be fatal. According to the Centers for Disease Control and Prevention, approximately 58 people die each year from bee, wasp or hornet stings. Emergency care for an insect sting includes immediately retreating to a safe location, away from where the sting occurred. You should then determine whether a stinger is still present at the sting site. If it is, you can scrape it off with a credit card. You should not attempt to remove it with a tweezers, since squeezing the stinger may inject additional venom into the patient. If the individual does not know if they are allergic, you should monitor them closely. If they know that they are allergic, immediately call 911 and follow the emergency care treatment for anaphylaxis.

Terror in the Sky
Stinging insects are responsible for nearly 60 deaths every year, the majority from anaphylactic reactions. If you are with a patient who is having an anaphylactic reaction inflicted by an insect sting, your first priority will be to move the patient out of the environment that contains the stinging insects.

ANAPHYLAXIS
EMERGENCY CARE

Here's what you should do if you find yourself with a patient who is suffering from anaphylaxis:

- Like a stroke, the most important treatment you can provide for someone suffering an anaphylactic reaction is to make that phone call to 911.
- If your patient has a known allergy, they may have a prescribed epinephrine auto-injector. Assist the patient in finding their auto-injector and help them to follow the instructions for its use. The Mayo Clinic advises that if the patient believes that they've come into contact with their known allergen, treatment should be started even if the patient is not showing outward signs and symptoms. The reality is that the body could be moving toward massive vasodilation, even if outward signs such as hives or swelling of the lips have not yet become apparent. Treatments such as Benadryl should only be considered if the patient has exhausted their supply of epinephrine or if the patient has no auto-injector with them.
- Keep the patient calm, treat them for shock, and monitor their airway.

SNAKE BITES

The vast majority of snakes in the U.S. are nonvenomous. However, venomous snakes make their homes in every state other than Alaska and Hawaii. Examples of venomous North American snakes include water moccasins, copperheads, three coral snake species and multiple rattlesnake species. But unlike Hollywood thrillers where snakebites are almost instantly lethal, even if you or a loved one is bitten by one of these venomous species, it's unlikely to result in death. In fact, of the estimated 70,000 snakebites that occur in the U.S. per year, only 15 percent of those are from venomous snakes — and only half of those cases involve the snake injecting venom. The Centers for Disease Control and Prevention estimates that only five people die every year from venomous snakes. That said, venomous snake bites can cause permanent nerve and tissue damage when not treated with anti-venom.

Signs and Symptoms

- Severe pain and swelling at the site of the bite. These signs and symptoms may take up to an hour to appear for most species, and up to 8 hours for rattlesnake bites.
- A tingling feeling spreads from the site of the bite.
- The patient experiences vomiting, perspiration, weakness and anxiety.

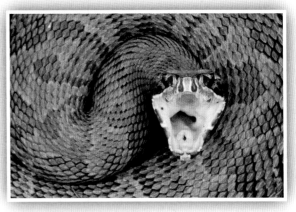

■ Water Moccasin

Habitat: Water moccasins live in the southeastern United States, from southern Virginia to Florida to eastern Texas. You will most likely find water moccasins swimming in swamps, marshes and drainage ditches and at the edges of ponds, lakes and streams.

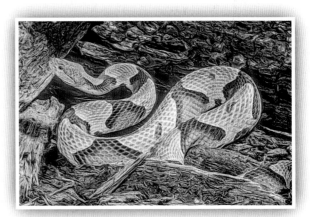

■ Copperhead

Habitat: Copperheads range from Massachusetts to Nebraska to Texas and much of the southeast United States. Copperheads tend to make heir homes in forested or rocky areas, although they can also inhabit wetlands.

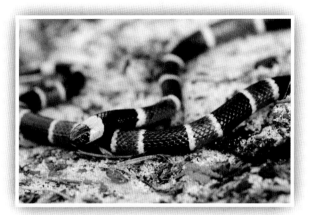

■ Coral Snake

Habitat: Coral snakes dwell in many southern states —
including most of Florida and from Louisiana through North
Carolina. Coral snakes tend to live in wooded, sandy and
marshy areas and will burrow underground.

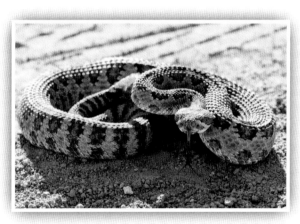

■ Rattlesnake

Habitat: With 7 of the top 10 most venomous snakes in
the U.S., rattlesnakes live in nearly every state and in a
variety of habitats. While they can be found in forests,
marshes, deserts and prairies, rattlesnakes tend to live in
open, rocky areas which offer them adequate prey and
protection from predators.

SNAKE BITE
EMERGENCY CARE

Here's what you should do if you find yourself
with a patient who was bitten by a snake that
you believe to be venomous:

- Wash the wound thoroughly with soap and
  water. Keep the bitten limb below the heart.
- Remove restrictive items such as rings.
- Bandage the wound with gauze and clear
  Tegaderm.
- While an ice pack would help to relieve
  discomfort, most EMS protocols advise
  against treating a venemous snakebite with
  ice. Some believe that applying ice would
  constrict the blood vessels, keeping the
  venom localized to the bite area and possibly
  leading to more significant nerve damage.
  That being said, there doesn't seem to be any
  published research to back up that opinion.
- Keep the patient calm and reassured. This
  helps to keep his or her heart rate low,
  slowing the spread of venom.
- Keep the patient from drinking caffeine or
  alcohol, which can speed the absorption rate
  of the venom.
- You should monitor the patient for signs and
  symptoms of an anaphylactic reaction.
- Under NO CIRCUMSTANCES should you cut
  into the snakebite and attempt to suction the
  venom from the wound nor apply a tourniquet
  in an attempt to slow the spread of venom.

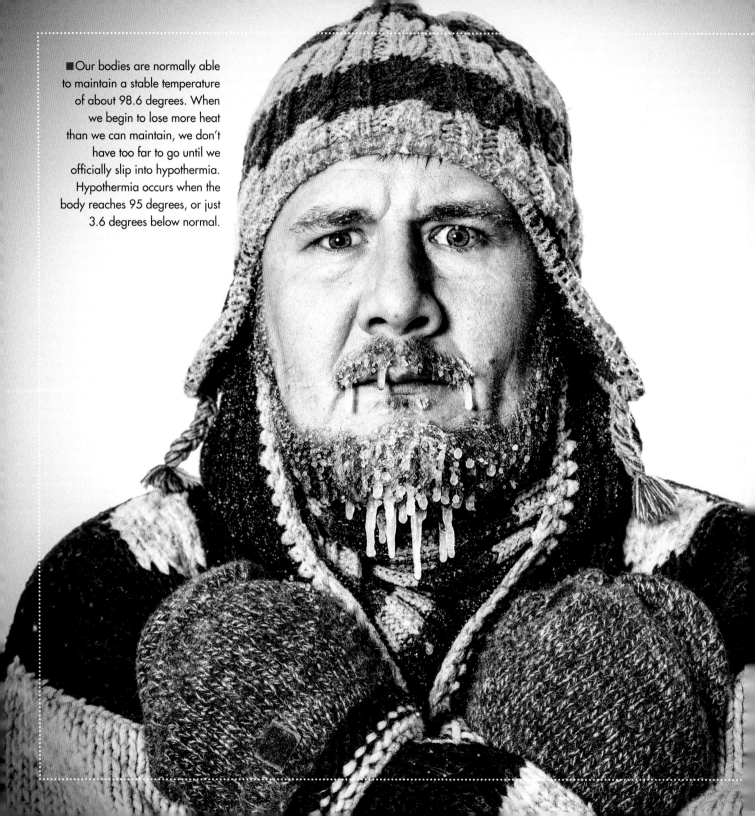

Our bodies are normally able to maintain a stable temperature of about 98.6 degrees. When we begin to lose more heat than we can maintain, we don't have too far to go until we officially slip into hypothermia. Hypothermia occurs when the body reaches 95 degrees, or just 3.6 degrees below normal.

ENVIRONMENTAL EMERGENCIES

The human body is normally able to regulate a stable temperature of about 98.6 degrees through metabolism, shivering and sweating. However, environmental conditions can cause the body to lose more heat than it can produce or take on more heat than it can dissipate. If either of those two conditions persist, the body will slip into hypothermia or hyperthermia, respectively. If this imbalance is not corrected quickly, the patient risks almost certain death.

The fact is, our bodies are built for a very narrow window of survivability when it comes to core temperature. When our core temperature drops to 95 degrees, we have officially slipped into hypothermia. A core temperature a mere 10 degrees higher at 105 degrees moves us into severe hyperthermia. In both cases, we are heading toward death unless that temperature can quickly be brought under control. We'll start this section with a discussion of hypothermia.

Hypothermia

Hypothermia can occur even in environments as warm as 65 degrees. It can take mere minutes if a patient has become immersed in cold water. Amazingly, the body will actually lose heat 25 to 30 times faster in water than in air of the same temperature. The stages of hypothermia include:

Stage 1: Shivering. Shivering is the body's response to heat loss. However, shivering typically does not occur below a body temperature of 90 degrees.

Stage 2: Apathy and decreased muscle function. At this stage, the symptoms can sometimes be mistaken for intoxication.

Stage 3: Decreased level of responsiveness.

HYPOTHERMIA
EMERGENCY CARE

When treating a patient suffering from hypothermia, you will have three goals:
1. Prevent further heat loss.
2. Rewarm the patient as quickly and safely as possible.
3. Observe the patient closely for further complications, such as cardiac arrest.

To accomplish those goals, you should:
- Call 911 and immediately move the patient from the environment that lead to hypothermia into a heated environment.
- If the patient is in wet clothing, remove it.
- Actively warm the patient by using heat packs in the armpits, groin and chest. Do NOT immerse the patient in hot water.
- Cover the patient with warm blankets on top and beneath his or her body.
- Handle the patient gently. Rough handling can result in ventricular fibrillation, leading to cardiac arrest.

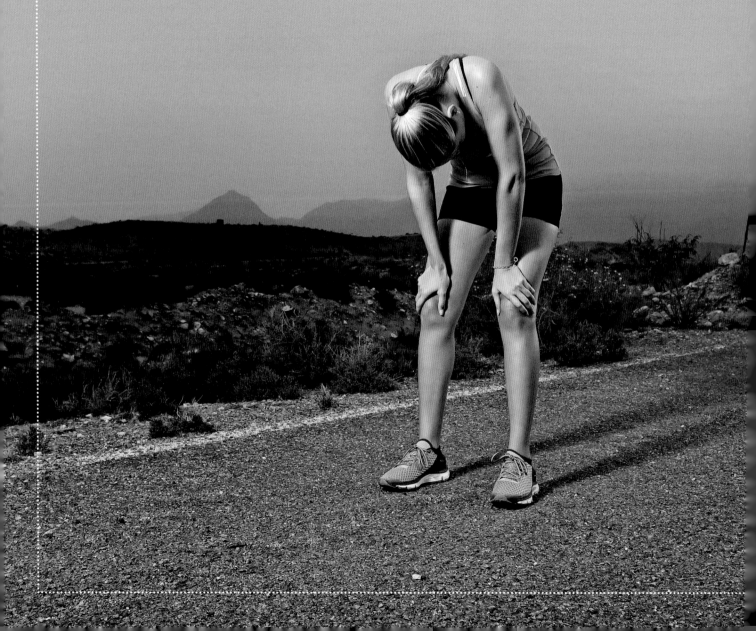

While we might tend to think of heat stroke as something that would only happen in an extreme environment, the condition can strike in even mild weather. Each year, thousands of athletes develop heat exhaustion and heat stroke, including more than 2,100 runners at the Boston Marathon in 2012. Temperatures didn't get above the upper 80s, yet one patient was admitted to an area hospital with an internal temperature of 108. Amazingly, she recovered.

Stage 4: Decreased vital signs, including a slow pulse and respiration rate.
Stage 5: Death.

Hyperthermia

Heat-related emergencies compose the category of hyperthermia and occur when the body is unable to dissipate as much heat as it is absorbing. Stages of hyperthermia include:

Heat Cramps

Heat cramps are muscle spasms or cramps caused by the loss of salt from the body through excessive sweating or from lactic acid buildup.

Heat Exhaustion

The next and more serious stage of hyperthermia is heat exhaustion. As the body works to dissipate heat in an extreme environment, it may cause prolonged sweating leading to large losses of water and salt. In addition, as the vessels dilate to bring heat to the surface of the skin and dissipate it through convection, blood is moved away from the major organs (including the brain), resulting in a mild case of shock.

Heat Stroke

The most serious stage of hyperthermia is heat stroke. This is a life-threatening emergency which occurs after the body loses its ability to further regulate its temperature, causing sweating to stop and the core temperature to continue to climb. Heat stroke is fatal in 20 to 80 percent of cases.

When treating a patient for heat stroke, cooling the patient takes priority over everything — other than the ABCs.

HEAT STROKE
EMERGENCY CARE

When treating a patient suffering from heat stroke, cooling the patient takes priority over everything — other than the ABCs.

Patient care should include the following:
- Call 911 and immediately move the patient into a cooled environment away from the environment that led to heat stroke.
- Remove as much of the patient's clothing as possible.
- Actively cool the patient by pouring tepid water over his or her body and by placing cold packs in the patient's armpits, on the sides of the neck, on the back of the knees, and in the groin.
- Monitor the patient for complicating factors such as seizures.

CHOKING

According to the National Safety Council, choking is the fourth leading cause of unintentional death. The bulk of these deaths occur among the very young and the very old. Among adults, food is the most common culprit while infants and toddlers often choke on foreign objects such as small toy parts. Choking occurs when an object becomes lodged in the trachea (the windpipe), blocking the flow of air to the lungs and the flow of oxygen to the brain. This leads to hypoxia and death unless the object is removed or dislodged.

Signs and Symptoms:
- Hands clutched to the throat, with a panicked look
- Inability to speak, cough or call out, indicating no air movement in or out
- Cyanosis
- Loss of consciousness

Field Treatment

To clear airway obstructions, the American Heart Association, the American Red Cross and most EMS protocols recommend a series of progressively aggressive steps designed to apply increasingly greater pressure to dislodge the blockage. Most guidelines recommend first encouraging the victim to cough, followed by back blows, followed by abdominal thrusts or chest thrusts.

Red Cross Guidelines

The Red Cross recommends alternating back blows with abdominal thrusts, in what they describe as a "five-and-five" approach:
- First, deliver **five back blows** between the person's shoulder blades with the heel of your hand.
- Then, perform **five abdominal thrusts**.
- Continue to alternate between five back blows and five abdominal thrusts until you dislodge the blockage.

American Heart Association Guidelines

For adults and children, the American Heart Association recommends abdominal thrusts without the back blows.

Heimlich Maneuver

Abdominal thrusts, also called the "Heimlich Maneuver" in deference to Henry J. Heimlich, a thoracic surgeon who developed the procedure in 1974, is used to dislodge airway obstructions by applying pressure on the bottom of the diaphragm to effectively produce an artificial cough.

Performing abdominal thrusts involves a rescuer standing behind a patient and using his or her hands to exert pressure on the bottom of the diaphragm. This compresses the lungs and exerts pressure on any object lodged in the trachea, hopefully expelling it.

It's important to know that even when performed properly, abdominal thrusts can cause injury to the choking victim. This includes potential damage to the xiphoid process, ribs, or internal organs including the diaphragm. For this reason, it's extremely important to only use abdominal thrusts when there is no air

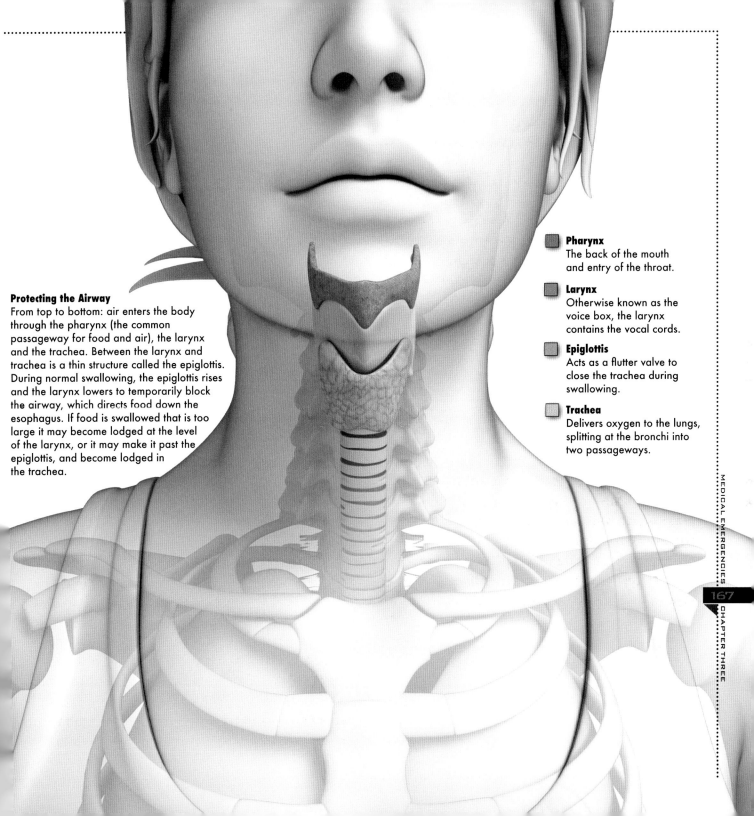

Protecting the Airway

From top to bottom: air enters the body through the pharynx (the common passageway for food and air), the larynx and the trachea. Between the larynx and trachea is a thin structure called the epiglottis. During normal swallowing, the epiglottis rises and the larynx lowers to temporarily block the airway, which directs food down the esophagus. If food is swallowed that is too large it may become lodged at the level of the larynx, or it may make it past the epiglottis, and become lodged in the trachea.

Pharynx
The back of the mouth and entry of the throat.

Larynx
Otherwise known as the voice box, the larynx contains the vocal cords.

Epiglottis
Acts as a flutter valve to close the trachea during swallowing.

Trachea
Delivers oxygen to the lungs, splitting at the bronchi into two passageways.

movement. If your patient is able to communicate with you (even if it's to say, "I'm choking, do something you idiot!"), that's enough of an indication that air is continuing to be exchanged. Back blows should be used in lieu of abdominal thrusts in such cases. When no air exchange is occurring, you should follow the procedures demonstrated on the opposite page.

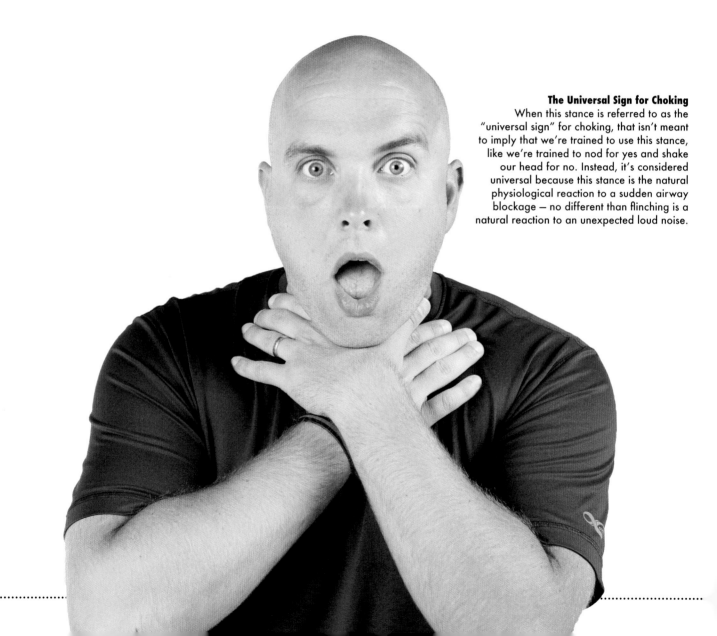

The Universal Sign for Choking
When this stance is referred to as the "universal sign" for choking, that isn't meant to imply that we're trained to use this stance, like we're trained to nod for yes and shake our head for no. Instead, it's considered universal because this stance is the natural physiological reaction to a sudden airway blockage — no different than flinching is a natural reaction to an unexpected loud noise.

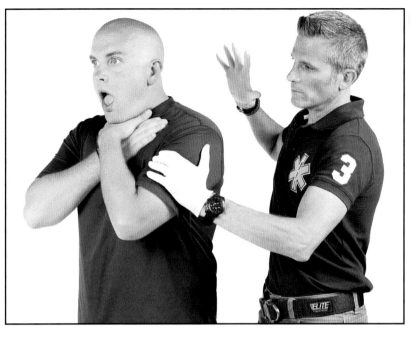

1 **Step 1:** If following the Red Cross guidelines, perform five back blows. If you have not dislodged the blockage, continue to step 2.

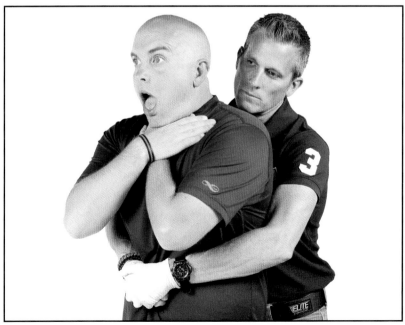

2 **Step 2:** Stand behind the patient. Wrap your arms around the waist and tip the person s lightly forward.

3 **Step 3:** Make a fist with one hand and position it between the patient's navel and the bottom of his sternum (the xiphoid process).

4 **Step 4:** Grasp the fist with your other hand. Press hard into the abdomen with a quick, upward thrust, as if trying to lift the person up. If the blockage is not dislodged, repeat the five-and-five cycle.

UNDERSTANDING SHOCK

Properly defined, shock is called **hypoperfusion**, which is a fancy way of saying that the body's cells are not receiving adequate oxygen, glucose and other nutrients. This is largely caused by an interruption in the body's transport system for those nutrients — namely the blood stream. The underlying cause might be serious arterial bleeding, anaphylactic reaction to a bee sting or massive fluid loss caused by third-

HYPOPERFUSION
[hipe-o-per-**few**-zhun]
An inadequate bloodstream delivery of oxygen, glucose and other nutrients to the body's cells.

degree burns. Regardless of the cause, you must not only treat the underlying condition to the best of your ability, you must also aggressively protect your patient from the effects of shock. Unless treated, shock will progress through three stages.

Stages of Shock

Compensatory Shock: As pressure drops inside the blood vessels, either due to blood loss or because the vessels have dilated (widened), the body compensates by releasing hormones in an attempt to constrict blood vessels and increase heart rate, thereby increasing blood pressure. During this stage, your patient may have normal blood pressure and an increased heart rate.

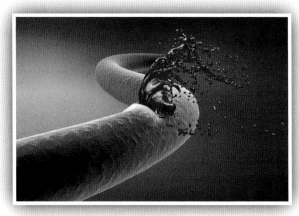

■ Hypovolemic Shock

The most common type of shock, caused by low blood volume or fluid loss. This might be caused by internal or external bleeding, plasma loss inflicted by severe burns, or it might be the result of fluid loss from severe dehydration or infection.

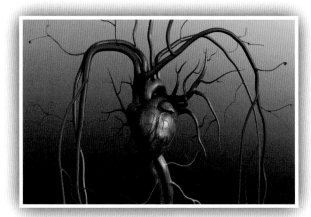

■ Cardiogenic Shock

Caused by a failure of the heart, which leads to decreased blood flow and blood pressure. In cardiogenic shock, there is no loss of blood volume and the vessels are properly dilated, but hypoperfusion occurs because the heart beats ineffectively. This may be the result of a heart attack, an infection, congestive heart failure (CHF) or another cause.

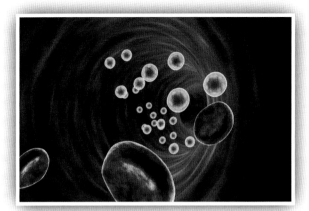

■ Vasogenic Shock

Caused by the rapid dilation (widening) of the vessels, possibly caused by a severe anaphylactic reaction. During vasogenic shock, there is no actual loss of blood or fluid from the vessels, but simply a larger volume of vessels for the same amount of blood. This results in a dramatic decrease in blood pressure, resulting in hypoperfusion.

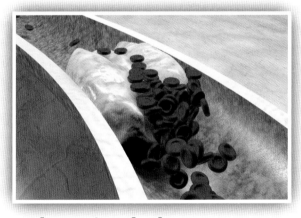

■ Obstructive Shock

Caused by a blockage of the blood stream, such as a clot or a pulmonary embolism (a clot that has lodged in the lung, and restricts the flow of blood returning to the heart). May also be caused by a tension pneumothorax, which puts pressure on the heart, reducing cardiac output.

SHOCK
EMERGENCY CARE

Any field treatment for shock has one underlying goal — to improve the delivery of oxygen and glucose to the brain and other cells.

To accomplish those goals, you should:

- Call 911 and immediately treat (if possible) any underlying condition that caused the patient to go into shock, such as stopping severe arterial bleeding.
- Since shock can compromise the body's ability to maintain a stable temperature, you should help to maintain body temperature by removing any wet clothing and covering the patient in a blanket.
- While elevating the patient's legs had been an accepted treatment for many years, that treatment has now fallen out of favor with many EMS agencies.
- Reassure the patient and monitor his or her airway.
- Assess the patient's breathing rate and quality. For patients with no breathing or inadequate rate or volume, begin rescue breaths.

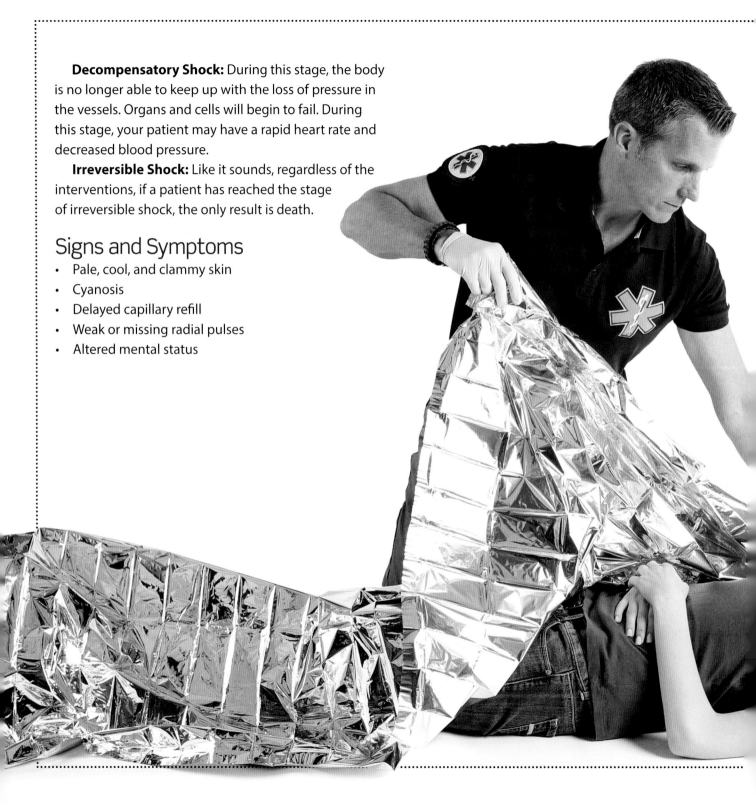

Decompensatory Shock: During this stage, the body is no longer able to keep up with the loss of pressure in the vessels. Organs and cells will begin to fail. During this stage, your patient may have a rapid heart rate and decreased blood pressure.

Irreversible Shock: Like it sounds, regardless of the interventions, if a patient has reached the stage of irreversible shock, the only result is death.

Signs and Symptoms

- Pale, cool, and clammy skin
- Cyanosis
- Delayed capillary refill
- Weak or missing radial pulses
- Altered mental status

Field Treatment

Any field treatment for shock has one underlying goal, which is to improve the delivery of oxygen and glucose to the brain and other cells. To do so, follow the field treatment outlined earlier. As a side note, you'll notice that I mentioned that elevating a patient's legs as a treatment for shock has fallen out of favor with many EMS agencies. Historically, the belief had been that elevating a patient's legs 8 to 12 inches provided more blood flow to the heart and brain, ultimately delivering more oxygen and glucose to the brain cells. However, a number of studies have concluded that the "shock position" does not provide any measurable positive effect on patient outcome. There has even been a concern that elevating the legs can increase intracranial pressure or make breathing more difficult for a patient who is already in distress. Instead, follow the treatments as outlined and aggressively treat (if possible) the underlying condition that led to shock. While you won't be able to reverse a pulmonary embolism, you will be able to stop severe bleeding, prevent a tension pneumothorax, and treat a severely burned patient with the right knowledge, the right tools, and the right confidence.

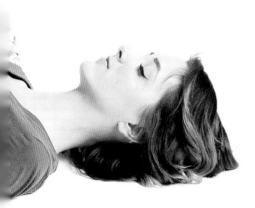

Maintaining Body Temperature
Since shock can compromise the body's ability to maintain a stable temperature, you should help to maintain body temperature by removing any wet clothing and covering the patient in a blanket.

→CHAPTER 4

BUILDING YOUR OWN FIRST-AID KIT

We've had a chance to review some amazing life-saving gear in Chapters 1, 2 and 3. But before you whip out the credit card and put in your order, consider two more items that are *more* important than any gadget. They are mindset and training.

Having the proper *mindset* will allow you to step into a leadership role when others falter. It will allow you to see past broken bones, spurting blood and hysterical bystanders and to focus on the task at hand. Ongoing *training*, especially hands-on training, will allow you to not only become fluid in your rapid assessment of a situation and of a patient, it will also allow you to confidently and *competently* implement the required treatments or tools. It also allows you to achieve those "MacGyver" moments when a field-expedient answer is the only solution. Gear is a distant priority after mindset and training.

I hope that this book has helped to set you on the path to a proper mindset, and we'll close this chapter with a discussion on training, so let's talk about the gear. There are a number of diagnostic tools, medications and devices accessible to EMS providers that are simply not available to nonprofessionals. However, the vast majority of the items that you'd find in a typical ambulance or medic bag (and the tools that were discussed in Chapters 1, 2 and 3) are things that nonprofessionals can find online with just a few clicks. Some you can even purchase at your local drugstore. To help prioritize your purchases, I'm going to suggest what type of gear *might* be included in emergency first-aid kits of three different sizes and roles. I'm also going to review a special kind of emergency first-aid kit, the Individual First-Aid Kit (IFAK). I'm a huge fan of IFAKs, which are better known as trauma kits. I'll also review a few pieces of gear that didn't make it into the previous chapters but which I include in my own

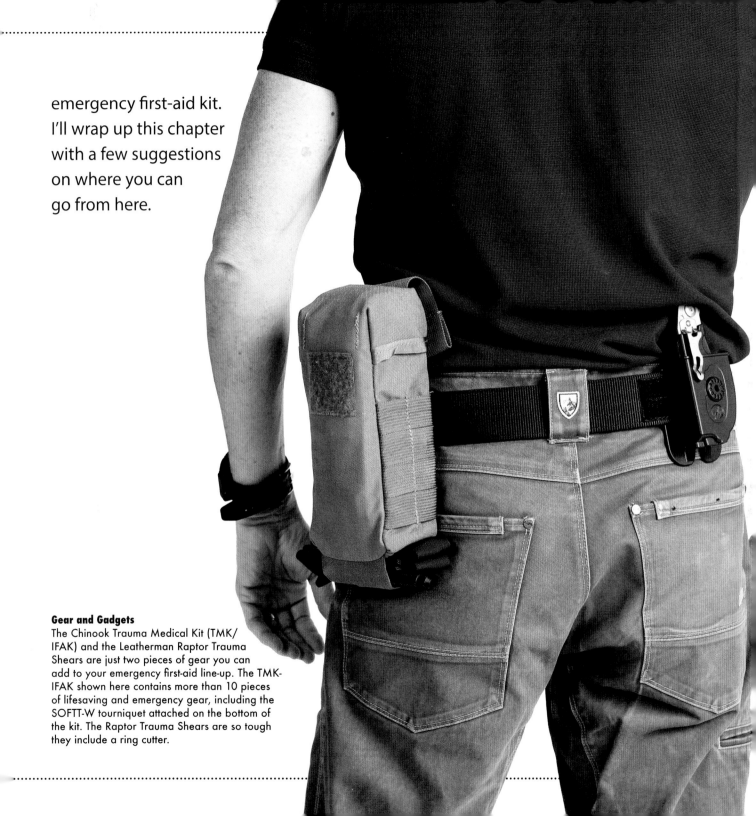

emergency first-aid kit.
I'll wrap up this chapter
with a few suggestions
on where you can
go from here.

Gear and Gadgets
The Chinook Trauma Medical Kit (TMK/
IFAK) and the Leatherman Raptor Trauma
Shears are just two pieces of gear you can
add to your emergency first-aid line-up. The TMK-
IFAK shown here contains more than 10 pieces
of lifesaving and emergency gear, including the
SOFTT-W tourniquet attached on the bottom of
the kit. The Raptor Trauma Shears are so tough
they include a ring cutter.

BUY OR BUILD?

A legitimate question to ask when planning out an emergency first-aid kit is, "Why not just buy a kit instead of building one?" That's a great question. The truth is, there are a lot of prepackaged emergency first-aid kits available. But, like buying a home versus building one — when you buy, you're buying a product that was built for someone else's needs, not yours. In addition, it's my personal belief that most prepackaged options (in particular, those you'd find at sporting goods or outdoors stores) focus far too heavily on "comfort items" rather than high-quality lifesaving items. It's also my belief that most of these kits are stocked with products designed to keep the price down. For example, while you might find a stack of 4x4 gauze in a prepackaged kit, you're unlikely to find an emergency bandage or an "H" bandage. You'll find "after bite" wipes and moleskin, but not an SOFTT-W or RMT tourniquet. You'll definitely find Band-Aids and triple antibiotic ointment, but you're unlikely to find a NuMask, adhesive sutures or benzoin swabs. So my preference is to build versus buy — even knowing that my homegrown kit will cost more than a prepackaged kit — because my kit will have *exactly* what I need in it and *nothing* that I don't need.

Before you buy a single product to go into your own emergency first-aid kit, you must answer one important, individual question. It's not one that can be answered by a company packing kits on the other side of the country in mass quantities. Ask yourself, "What's the mission?" In other words, in what environment and what capacity do you want the emergency first-aid kit to serve? Your "mission" will change depending upon where you are or where you'll be; what you'll be doing; who you'll be supporting; and how far from EMS coverage you are.

The reality is, you might require more than one kit. Alternatively, your kit might need to be unpacked and repacked with different supplies depending upon your plans. For example, if you want an emergency first-aid kit that can deal with the most probable emergencies that might occur during a weekend car camping trip in the suburbs, your kit should contain different items and be of a different size than a kit designed to support a week-long hunting trip hours from cell phone and EMS coverage. While your needs may be different than mine, I'm going to provide a suggested *starting* point for what might go into small, medium and large kits. Based upon your particular "mission," you can choose to add items or remove items from my list. One last suggestion is to unpack and repack your kit(s) frequently to become intimately familiar with the supplies you've chosen. This also gives you an opportunity to find out when something is missing. At my department, we'll inventory our ambulance supplies and medic bags at the start and end of every shift. Not only does that help to identify what (if anything) is missing and needs resupply, but it also builds muscle memory to know *exactly* where everything is.

Comfort Versus Lifesaving

Regardless of the size of the kit, I like to categorize items by whether they're a "comfort" item or a life-sustaining item. Comfort items are found in most first-aid kits and would include things such as Band-Aids, first-aid cream, poison ivy wipes, aspirin and cold packs. That said, many "comfort" items can become life-sustaining items in the proper situation. For example, as discussed in Chapter 3, aspirin can provide a life-sustaining boost to individuals who are suffering chest pains caused by a heart attack (but who have not yet moved into cardiac arrest). Cold packs can be used to comfort a patient who has suffered a broken ankle or wrist. You can also save the life of a heat stroke patient by placing ice packs on the major blood vessels on the neck, armpits and groin. On my suggested list of items, I've placed those multitalented items in the "Comfort Items" list.

Small Kit Contents

Let's start by creating a small emergency first-aid kit. This is the type of kit that you'd take with you when EMS is no more than 10 minutes away. In other words, when you're fully under the EMS umbrella. It will include a handful of comfort items and a few lifesaving items.

Comfort Items

- Individual packs or a bottle of Benadryl
- Individual packs or a bottle of baby aspirin
- 10 Band-Aids
- 10 alcohol preps
- Triple antibiotic ointment
- Tweezers
- Moleskin
- Small Tegaderm gel bandage
- 1 pack of compressed gauze
- 2 pairs of nitrile gloves

Lifesaving Items

- Two 4x4 surgical sponges
- 25-gram QuikClot sponge
- Tourniquet
- Oral rehydration salts

Medium Kit Contents

Next, let's step up to a medium-sized kit. This is the kind of kit you'd take with you when EMS is no farther than an hour away — such as during a day hike.

Comfort Items

- Individual packs or a bottle of Benadryl
- Individual packs or a bottle of baby aspirin
- 20 Band-Aids of various size
- 20 alcohol preps
- Triple antibiotic ointment
- Tweezers
- Moleskin
- 1 small and 1 large Tegaderm gel bandage
- 1 pack of compressed gauze
- 4 pairs of nitrile gloves
- 36-inch SAM splint
- Triangular bandage
- Self-adhering bandage wrap
- 2 packets of poison ivy toxin removal cloths
- 1 instant cold pack

Lifesaving Items
- Four 4x4 surgical sponges
- "H" or emergency bandage
- 25-gram QuikClot sponge
- Medium-sized burn dressing
- Pocket mask or NuMask
- Tourniquet
- Oral rehydration salts
- Trauma shears

Large Kit Contents

Finally, let's talk about what might go into a large kit. This is the kind of kit you'd take with you when EMS is farther than a day away, such as on a multi-day backpacking or canoeing trip. This kit can be as large as you're willing to carry, but at a minimum, you should include the following items:

Comfort Items
- Bottle of Benadryl
- Bottle of baby aspirin
- 30 Band-Aids of various size
- 30 alcohol preps
- Triple-antibiotic ointment
- Tweezers
- Moleskin
- Multiple Tegaderm gel bandages of various size
- 36-inch, 18-inch, 9-inch and finger SAM splints
- 2 triangular bandages
- 2 packs of compressed gauze
- 10 pairs of nitrile gloves
- 2 rolls of self-adhering bandage wrap
- 4 packets of poison ivy toxin removal cloths
- 4 instant cold packs

Lifesaving Items
- Ten 4x4 surgical sponges
- 2 "H" or emergency bandages
- Two 25-gram QuikClot sponges
- 100-gram QuikClot sponge
- Large-sized burn dressing
- Pocket mask or NuMask
- Bottle of wound cleaning spray or sterile water and povidone-iodine foil pack
- Large volume syringe
- Vented chest seal
- Tourniquet
- 4 packets of 3M Steri-Strips
- Oral rehydration salts
- Large trauma pad
- Trauma shears
- Emergency blanket
- Eye shield

As mentioned, consider these gear lists as a starting point for your own various-sized kits. Adjust the contents to fit your own particular needs. Since it may be difficult to visualize just how much gear this actually entails, the following pages should give you a good visual of how large a pack might be needed to carry this amount of gear. I've also included a bit of extra commentary on some of the specific brands that I've grown to count on.

PURCHASING SUPPLIES

When creating your own kit, you'll discover that your local drugstore can provide quite a few of the basic products. For more advanced products (the types of things that rarely show up in prepackaged kits), go directly to one of the EMS suppliers. My personal favorites are Chinook Medical (ChinookMed.com) out of Durango, Colorado, and Rescue Essentials (Rescue-Essentials.com) out of Salida, Colorado. As you browse those websites, keep in mind that just because you can buy decompression needles, skin staplers or suture kits, doesn't mean that they're right for *you*. Unless you've had proper training with such devices, you risk making a bad situation, worse. Always operate within your level of training, but keep in mind that many of the products discussed and demonstrated in this book are products that you can learn to use effectively through self-led, hands-on training. That may mean purchasing a spare of those products (one to train with, one to keep sterile and packaged), but the extra investment will be worth it. The time to learn how to use your "H" bandage or RMT tourniquet is *not* when a companion has blood spurting from a lacerated brachial artery.

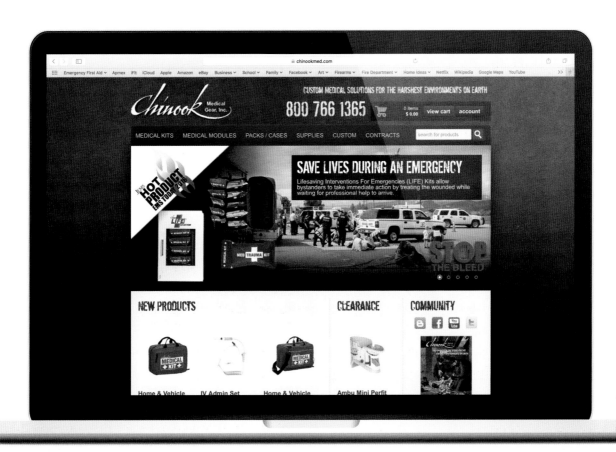

Chinook Medical
Chinook Medical is one of my favorite online resources. Not only because they've developed some amazing trauma kits, but also because they have a narrow focus on the type of gear that belongs in emergency first-aid kits. They don't clutter their website with hundreds of other products. Chinook Medical is veteran-owned and has an incredibly responsive staff to help you with your purchases.

1 ▪ H&H COMPRESSED GAUZE

Takes up about 1/4 of the space needed for a traditional roll of gauze such as Kerlix. If you trim off the edges of the vacuum pack, it will pack even smaller. See the "Additional Gear and Gadgets" section later in this chapter to learn more. MSRP: $2.44

2 ▪ NUMASK

As mentioned in Chapter 1, the NuMask is an alternative to the traditional pocket mask. It is designed to create a better seal by operating more like a snorkel than a mask. Another big plus is that it is much smaller than a pocket mask and can easily fit into a small emergency first-aid kit, your glove box or a purse.
MSRP: $17.50 WITH CASE

3 ▪ RMT TOURNIQUET

While any of the tourniquets reviewed in Chapter 2 will work, the Ratcheting Medical Tourniquet (RMT) is so easy to use that it makes a great choice for a small kit. But, just because it's easy to use, doesn't mean that it requires no practice. MSRP: $33.00

4 ▪ BABY ASPIRIN & BENADRYL

When you're under the umbrella of EMS, you don't need to include a lot of meds in your kit. However, since both aspirin and Benadryl fill multiple needs, they're a good addition to any sized kit. Depending upon your pack size, you can squeeze in small bottles or choose individual packets. Benadryl is a brand name; you'll find the individual packets under the name diphenhydramine.

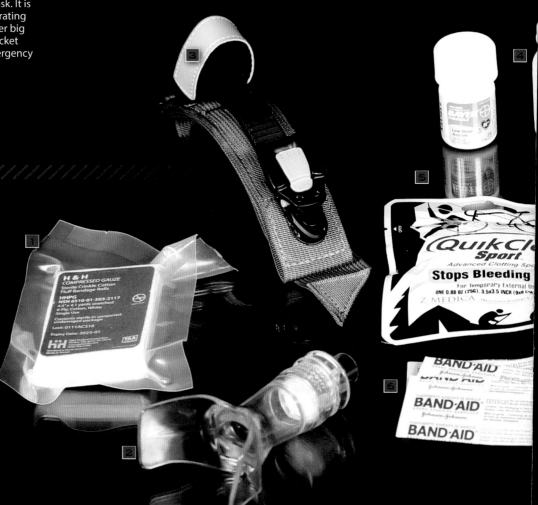

5 ■ QUIKCLOT SPONGE

Even without a compression bandage to hold it down, a hemostatic dressing like QuikClot can stop severe bleeding. Place it on the injury and provide direct pressure. Just don't forget to wear your nitrile gloves.
MSRP: $14.95 FOR A 25-GRAM SPONGE

6 ■ BAND-AIDS AND MOLESKIN

I mentioned that prepackaged emergency first-aid kits often focus too heavily on comfort items like Band-Aids, but I've seen the opposite occur as well. Some full-sized packs have every lifesaving device imaginable, but lack basic boo-boo fixing products such as bandages, moleskin and triple-antibiotic ointment.
MSRP: VARIES

7 ■ TEGADERM GEL BANDAGE

Tegaderm gel bandages fill a lot of roles including covering scrapes, lacerations or minor burns. Even in your smallest kit, these paper-thin products can find a corner to squeeze into. These come in a wide variety of sizes.
MSRP: $19.00 FOR 10 COUNT OF 6X8

8 ■ GAUZE SPONGES

Great for handling everything from a severe arterial bleed to wiping dirt and gravel out of a skinned knee.
MSRP: $5.45 FOR A BOX OF 50

9 ■ UNCLE BILL'S TWEEZERS

Not every tweezer deserves its own storage cylinder or keychain, but Uncle Bill's does. Made in Hartford, Connecticut, these tweezers have perfectly aligned precision tips, — better than anything out there. General Norman Schwarzkopf used a pair during Desert Storm and said, "I have never had a pair of tweezers in my life that was worth a damn. Now I do and I appreciate it very much." **MSRP: $6.99**

10 ■ ORAL REHYDRATION SALTS

While water or a Gatoraid can work in a pinch to rehydrate you or a companion, these oral rehydration salts are designed to rebalance an out-of-whack system. The pack is small enough to fit at least one into even the smallest kit.
MSRP: $1.35 FOR SINGLE UNIT

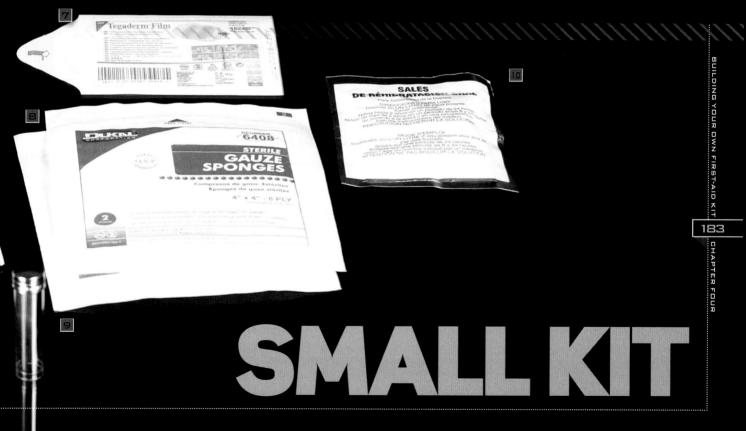

SMALL KIT

1 ■ INSTANT COLD PACKS

In a medium-sized kit, you won't be able to pack enough cold packs to make a significant difference to a heat stroke victim, but one pack will bring comfort to someone who has suffered a strain, sprain or fracture. The biggest issue with cold packs are their size and fragile nature. While you can jam an "H" or emergency bandage into the corner of your pack, if you do that with an ice pack, you'll end up with a ruined ice pack, and a first-aid kit full of ammonium nitrate beads. Maybe someday H&H will develop a compressed cold pack the same size as their compressed gauze. MSRP: $1.00

2 ■ POISON IVY WIPES

If you're with a companion who only packed an IFAK trauma kit and they wade into poison ivy, they'll trade everything in their kit for one poison ivy wipe. Premoistened with urushiol — an agent designed to bind with the toxin in poison ivy. MSRP: $19.99 FOR A BOX OF 6.

3 ■ BURN DRESSING

As discussed in Chapter 2, second- and third-degree burns that cover less than 9 percent of the body can be treated with gel-based dressings, which will cool the burn and relieve pain. These 4x4 dressings by Water-Jel Technologies are meant for small burns, but Water-Jel burn produces dressings as large as 11x19, as well as specialty dressings for burned hands and facial burns. MSRP: $3.83

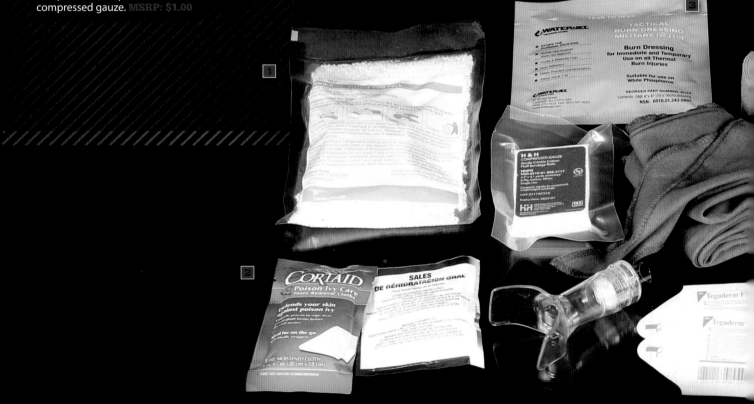

4 ▪ 36-INCH SAM SPLINT

As demonstrated in Chapter 2, the innovative uses for SAM splints in treating strains, sprains and fractures are as limitless as your imagination. In a medium kit, pack at least one 36-inch splint which you can purchase either rolled or folded flat. Of course, since it's infinitely flexible, you can mold it into whatever shape you want to fit it in your kit. Also include a roll of self-adhering bandage wrap.
MSRP: $10.95

5 ▪ 3M STERI-STRIPS

While there are plenty of adhesive sutures on the market, the 3M Steri-Strips are a good bet because of their packaging. Other adhesive sutures are packed for hospital use in paper packaging, which easily rips when stuffed into a first-aid kit. Plus, if you need to use just one or two sutures, the paper packaged versions are impossible to reseal. Not so with the Steri-Strips, which ship in a tough resealable plastic envelope.
MSRP: $5.00 FOR A 10-STRIP ENVELOPE

6 ▪ "H" OR EMERGENCY COMPRESSION BANDAGE

If you can squeeze one into your small kit, do it. Otherwise, save it for a medium or large kit. My preference is for the "H" bandage, but the emergency bandage also has a phenomenal track record. **MSRP: $6.00**

7 ▪ TRAUMA SHEARS

Most large pre-packaged kits come with a rudimentary pair of trauma shears, but the pivot screw will most likely snap the first time you need to use them to cut more than paper. Spend the money to get a decent pair with a non-stick coating such as black-oxide or titanium nitride. Or, for a real game changer, check out my review on the Leatherman Raptor in the "Additional Gear and Gadgets" section later in this chapter.
MSRP: $11.00

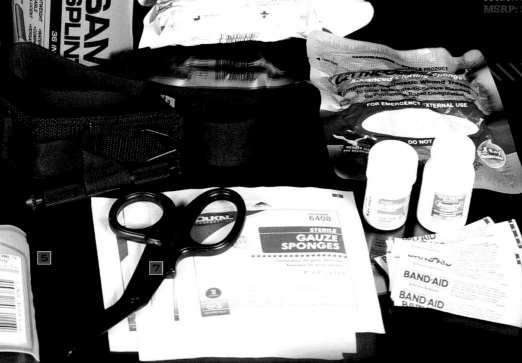

MEDIUM KIT

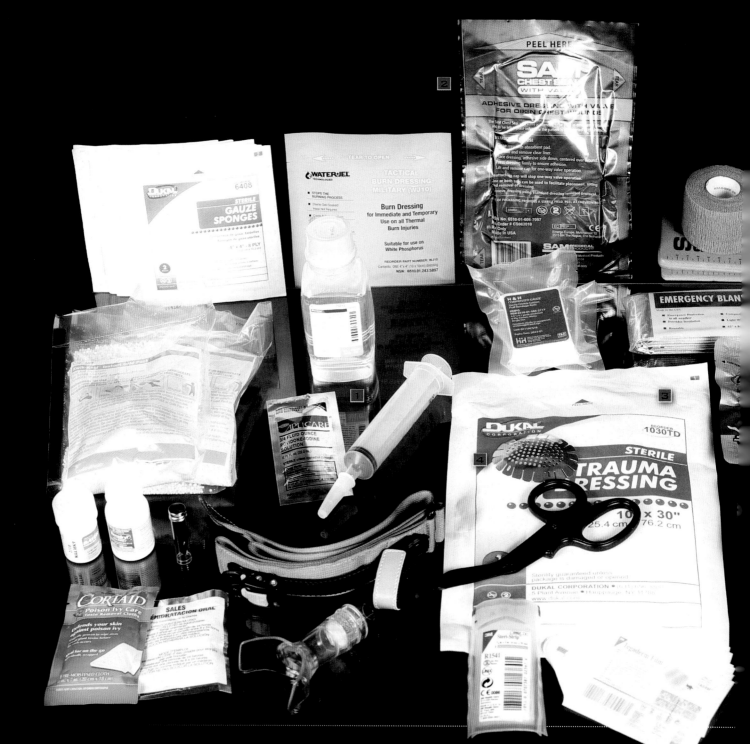

1 ◼ POVIDONE-IODINE FOIL PACK

While a wound can be cleaned using water that has been sterilized through boiling, a mixture of sterilized water and a povidone-iodine foil pack speeds the process and results in a more antiseptic environment to prevent infection.
MSRP: $2.36 FOR 5

2 ◼ SAM CHEST SEAL (VENTED)

The Bolin or Asherman vented chest seals have small enough valve profiles that they can be rolled and squeezed into a small or medium kit or even an IFAK. However, the larger valve profile on the SAM means it's really only going to fit in a larger kit. For a comparison of those three chest seals, see Chapter 2. MSRP: $22.50

3 ◼ LARGE TRAUMA DRESSING

You can think of a large trauma dressing as a gigantic surgical sponge. While a stack of 4x4 surgical sponges is an appropriate solution if you're applying direct pressure on a moderate arterial bleed, a large trauma dressing is meant for larger trauma. For large bleeds or third-degree burns covering *more* than 9 percent of the body, the trauma dressing should be placed dry. For abdominal eviscerations or burns covering *less* than 9 percent of the body, the dressing should be placed wet.
MSRP: $4.00 FOR A 10X30

4 ◼ FOX ALUMINUM EYE SHIELD

As demonstrated in Chapter 2, an eye shield can make all the difference when dealing with trauma to the eyeball. For an innovative alternative to holding an eye shield in place with gauze and self-adhering bandage wrap, see the "Additional Gear and Gadgets" section later in this chapter.
MSRP: $14.52 FOR A PACK OF 10

5 ◼ 9-, 18- AND 36-INCH SAM SPLINTS COMBO PACK

For a large kit, I suggest packing one or two of each size of SAM splint. The best deal I've found so far is from Rescue Essentials for a combo-pack of two splints in all three sizes, plus two finger splints and four rolls of black self-adhering bandage wrap.
MSRP: $46.49 FOR RESCUE ESSENTIALS' COMBO-PACK

6 ◼ EMERGENCY BLANKET

A sleeping bag will offer better insulation and warmth to a patient suffering from hypothermia or shock, but if that item has been left back at your campsite miles away, you'll appreciate having an emergency blanket in your kit.
MSRP: $1.57

LARGE KIT

TRAUMA KITS

I spent the previous few pages extolling the virtues of the "build-your-own" approach to creating emergency first-aid kits. But I have to admit that I've become a big fan of one particular type of prepackaged kit: the Individual First-Aid Kit (IFAK). The name doesn't come close to describing the lifesaving tools packed into these kits. More appropriately, IFAK are also known as Individual Trauma Kits. Fitting, since the kits are meant to provide several devices designed to save a patient from life-threatening trauma. "Individual" doesn't just refer to their small size — they are meant to be worn on the belt or gear attachments of the kit owner. If a traumatic emergency occurs, the rescuers would use the IFAK worn on the victim — the individual — not their own kit. Developed on the battlefields of Iraq and Afghanistan, these kits have now entered the civilian market through companies like Dark Angel, Chinook Medical and others.

Trauma kits are not your everyday first-aid kit. You won't find comfort items such as moleskin, Band-Aids or "after-bite" wipes. Instead, the kits are designed to provide immediate access to the lifesaving tools necessary for significant trauma, such as a devastating gunshot wound. Instead of thinking of the kits as a collection of tools, you can think of them as mitigation kits for specific life-threatening trauma including:

- Severe bleeding, which can quickly lead to decompensatory shock and death.
- An open pneumothorax, which can quickly lead to a tension pneumothorax and death.
- A compromised airway, which can quickly lead to hypoxia and death.

As with a more general emergency first-aid kit, you can build your own trauma kit and throw it in a pouch of your choosing. But as you'll see in the two IFAKs that I'll profile next, what makes the kits from Dark Angel and Chinook Medical unique isn't necessarily the gear (which you *can* buy on your own). What makes them unique are the pouches that *hold* the gear. Both the Dark Angel Gen 3 and the Chinook Medical TMK-IFAK are designed to deploy their life-saving devices *quickly*, without forcing a user to fumble with zippers or snaps. In fact, both pouches give you immediate access to a tourniquet by storing it on the outside of the pouch. Additionally, both allow you to literally rip the contents out of the pouch by pulling a deployment handle or strap. One second your IFAK is sealed up safe and secure in its pouch; the next second, you've got a chest seal, an emergency bandage and a tourniquet in your gloved hands.

One last comment on any IFAK: these are first-aid kits that are meant to be worn, not left in your hall closet at home. If you hunt, camp, backpack, kayak, climb mountains or visit your local gun range, you'll want an IFAK on your hip.

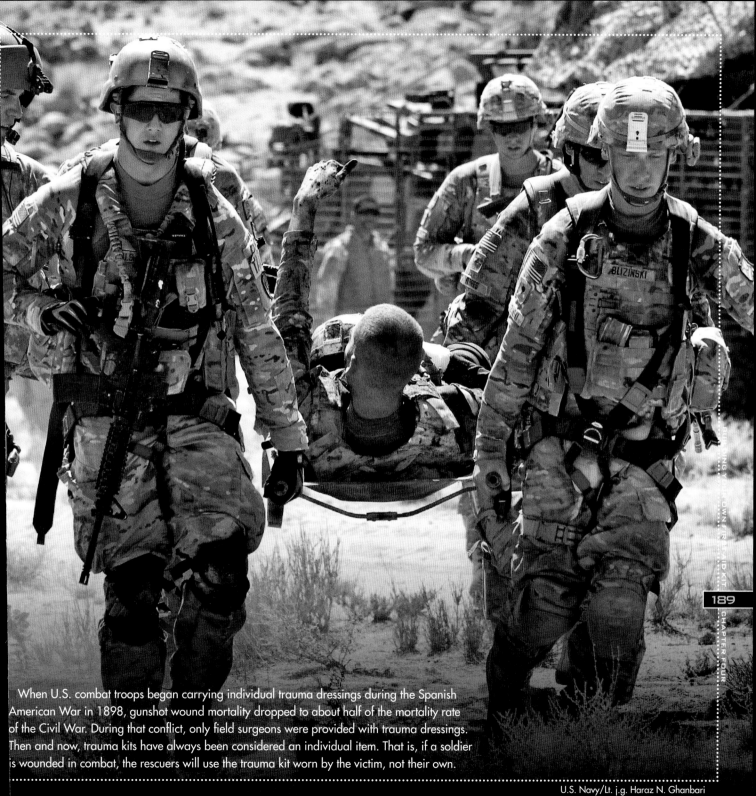

When U.S. combat troops began carrying individual trauma dressings during the Spanish American War in 1898, gunshot wound mortality dropped to about half of the mortality rate of the Civil War. During that conflict, only field surgeons were provided with trauma dressings. Then and now, trauma kits have always been considered an individual item. That is, if a soldier is wounded in combat, the rescuers will use the trauma kit worn by the victim, not their own.

U.S. Navy/Lt. j.g. Haraz N. Ghanbari

D.A.R.K. (DIRECT ACTION RESPONSE KIT) GEN 3 TRAUMA KIT
The Pouch and Contents

The D.A.R.K Gen 3 Trauma Kit is just one of several trauma kits available from Dark Angel Medical (DarkAngelMedical.com), but it's my favorite of their kits because of its size and easy access to two key devices — the tourniquet and trauma shears. Both are accessible externally without opening the kit. In its standard configuration, the Gen 3 contains:

- 1 Pair nitrile gloves, size Large
- 1 SOFTT tourniquet or 1 CAT tourniquet
- 2 HALO seals (contained in one package)
- 1 Nasopharyngeal airway
- 1 Israeli emergency bandage, 4-inch
- 1 QuikCLot Combat Gauze LE or CELOX Rapid (MIL-SPEC kits contain QuikClot Combat Gauze MIL)
- 1 Compressed gauze
- 1 Mylar blanket
- 1 Polycarbonate eyeshield (the current USMC-issue eye shield which is recommended by the Committee on Tactical Casualty Combat Care)
- 1 Ten Tac Med Tips assessment card

If selecting the MIL-SPEC configuration, the kit will also contain the following:
- 1 TCCC casualty documentation tool
- One 14-gauge ARS decompression needle

As mentioned earlier, unless you are trained in using a decompression needle, you should not select this configuration. The same is true for the nasal airway. Although it is included in the basic configuration, you should ignore it unless you've been trained to use it properly. However, don't discard those items if your kit happens to contain them. A rescuer with a higher level of training might be at the same scene — and may even need to use them on you. Dark Angel also allows you to choose between a CAT or SOFTT tourniquet (I personally prefer the SOFTT), and you may upgrade the standard shears to rip shears for an additional $24.95. The standard shears will cut through pant legs and shirts. The rip shears include a hook-knife on the grips and will do a superior job of cutting through leather jackets, belts and boots.

Unlike the TMK-IFAK from Chinook Medical, the D.A.R.K. Gen 3 vacuum packs all of its devices into a single package, which significantly reduces the space requirements. On the other hand, that means that once the vacuum pack is opened, you'll have to keep track of each item, and if your only need was for the compressed gauze, you're now stuck with a pile of items that will need to be vacuum packed again, in the same size and shape as the original package. That said, Dark Angel offers an innovative guarantee, which is that if you're ever required to deploy one of their kits to save a life, they'll ship you a refill at no charge. Considering the refill for the Gen 3 is $97.95, that's a pretty nice guarantee.

One final comment on the contents of the Gen 3. Dark Angel currently packs their kits with HALO non-vented chest seals. As discussed in Chapter 2, unless you are within minutes of EMS care, or unless an individual on the scene is trained in using a decompression needle to deal with a tension pneumothorax, I recommend using vented seals over non-vented seals. However, one significant benefit of the HALO seals is that they are packed two to a package, which is critical when dealing with an entry *and* an exit wound.

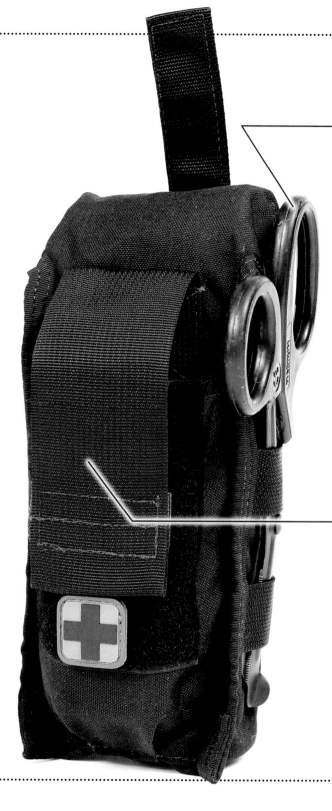

Trauma Shears
The Gen 3 stores its trauma shears on the exterior of the pouch, making them instantly accessible if you need to quickly cut away clothing that's masking a significant injury.

CAT or SOFTT Tourniquet
One of my favorite aspects of the Dark Angel Gen 3 is that the tourniquet is instantly available to you, as it's stored on the exterior of the pouch. Rip open the velcro tab for immediate access. Since the Gen 3 can be ordered with either a CAT or SOFTT, you must take the time to train with your tourniquet of choice. Although similar in design (they both use a windlass) they require different steps during deployment.

D.A.R.K. (DIRECT ACTION RESPONSE KIT) GEN 3 TRAUMA KIT

1. Emergency Bandage

As explained in Chapter 2, compression bandages such as the emergency bandage and the "H" bandage constitute must-haves in trauma kits. Buy an extra bandage so that you can practice with it until deploying it becomes second nature.

2. HALO Chest Seals (2)

HALO chest seals get top scores for adhesiveness, even when a chest is covered in blood and sweat. The pack contains two seals, which you will need if dealing with an entry and an exit wound. However, since HALO seals lack a vent, you must monitor your patient closely for signs of a tension pneumothorax (explained in Chapter 2) and "burp" the seal if those signs and symptoms develop.

3. QuikCLot Combat Gauze LE

The hemostatic agent in QuikClot Combat Gauze LE (or MIL) combined with the emergency bandage is all you need to mitigate all but the most severe bleeds. If those two items don't cut it, you can always jump up to the tourniquet, easily accessible on the outside of the pouch.

4. Nitrile Gloves

While you might wear a medium glove (as I do), most trauma kits are packed with large gloves because the gloves aren't necessarily designed to fit you. They're designed to fit the rescuer who is using your kit to save your life if you're the victim of a gunshot wound or other significant trauma.

5. Compressed Gauze

As you'll see in the next section, "Additional Gear and Gadgets," compressed gauze might look tiny in its vacuum-packed packaging, but once it's opened and unrolled, it contains an incredible amount of gauze — as much as is contained in a full roll of Kerlix. This gauze can be used when applying direct pressure to stem the flow of blood or to hold the eye shield in place.

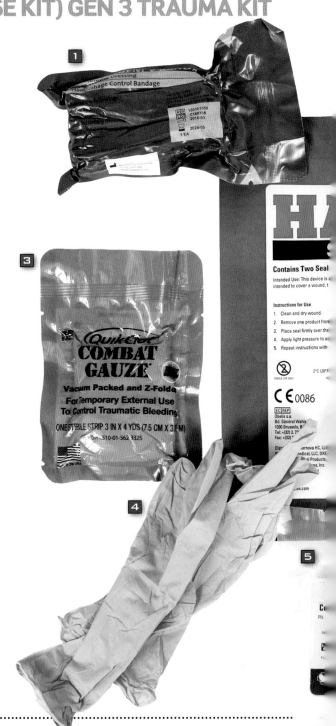

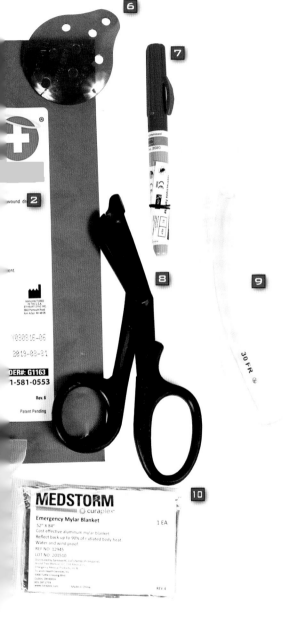

6. Polycarbonate Eye Shield
As outlined in Chapter 2, an eye shield is a critical part of treating severe eye trauma including an injured globe. After applying the shield, you can hold it in place with the gauze. If you've also packed self-sticking tape such as Coban or CoFlex, you can snug the gauze in place.

7. Decompression Needle
In the hands of a properly trained rescuer, a decompression needle can reduce the chances of a tension pneumothorax by venting off air that is becoming trapped in the pleural space due to a penetration of the chest. If you're not trained in its use, don't attempt to use it, but do let any rescuers with a higher level of training know that you have it. By the way, watching a video on YouTube doesn't count as training.

8. Trauma Shears
Like its tourniquet, the Gen 3 stores its trauma shears outside the pack for easy accessibility. My suggestion is to pay the $24.95 to upgrade from the standard shears to the rip shears.

9. Nasal Airway
Nasal airways should only be used by rescuers trained in their use. If you are trained, you should not hesitate to use it for a patient who has an altered mental status. If you're unsure of whether they have an altered mental status or whether they'll accept the airway, go ahead and attempt to insert it. The patient will remove any mystery real fast. Those who have been trained to employ a nasal airway will recall that its use is contraindicated when the patient has head trauma — in particular, when you suspect a basilar skull fracture.

10. Mylar Blanket
The mylar blanket wasn't in the original Gen 3 insert, and it was a brilliant addition. After treating your patient for severe bleeding or an open pneumothorax, don't forget to treat for shock by covering him or her with the blanket.

CHINOOK TRAUMA MEDICAL KIT (TMK-IFAK)
The Pouch and Contents

The TMK-IFAK (Trauma Medical Kit — Individual First-Aid Kit) from Chinook Medical is easily one of my favorites due to its innovative method of deployment, which I'll touch on it a moment. In its standard configuration, the TMK-IFAK contains:

- 1 Pair nitrile gloves, size large
- 1 SOFTT-W tourniquet or 1 CAT tourniquet
- 1 Compressed gauze
- 1 Israeli emergency bandage, 4-inch
- 1 Bolin chest seal
- One 14-gauge ARS decompression needle
- 1 Nasopharyngeal airway
- 1 Aluminum eye shield
- 1 Pair trauma shears, 5.5"
- 1 Permanent marker
- 1 Flat duct tape, 1.89" x 2 yards, OD
- 1 Tactical combat casualty care card

As with the Dark Angel kit, unless you are trained in using a decompression needle or nasal airway, you can simply ignore them during a traumatic emergency — or let a rescuer with the proper training know that you have them available. Chinook Medical also allows you to choose between a CAT or SOFTT-W tourniquet as you are configuring your kit.

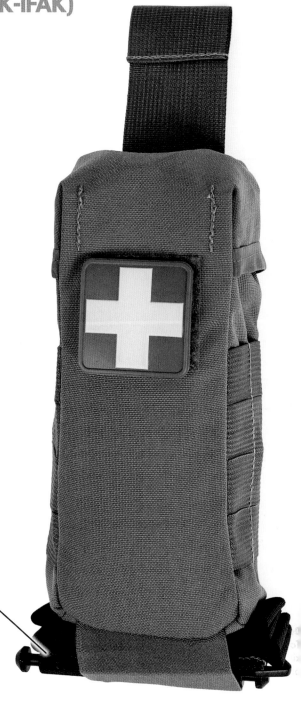

SOFTT-W Tourniquet

If you choose the tourniquet from SOF, you'll get the updated SOFTT-W tourniquet with its wider configuration (1.5 inches versus 1.0 inch) and its simple ability to disconnect the slip-gate buckle from the strap by twisting it free from the U-shaped clip. Doing so allows you to deploy the tourniquet on a limb which might be trapped under an immovable object.

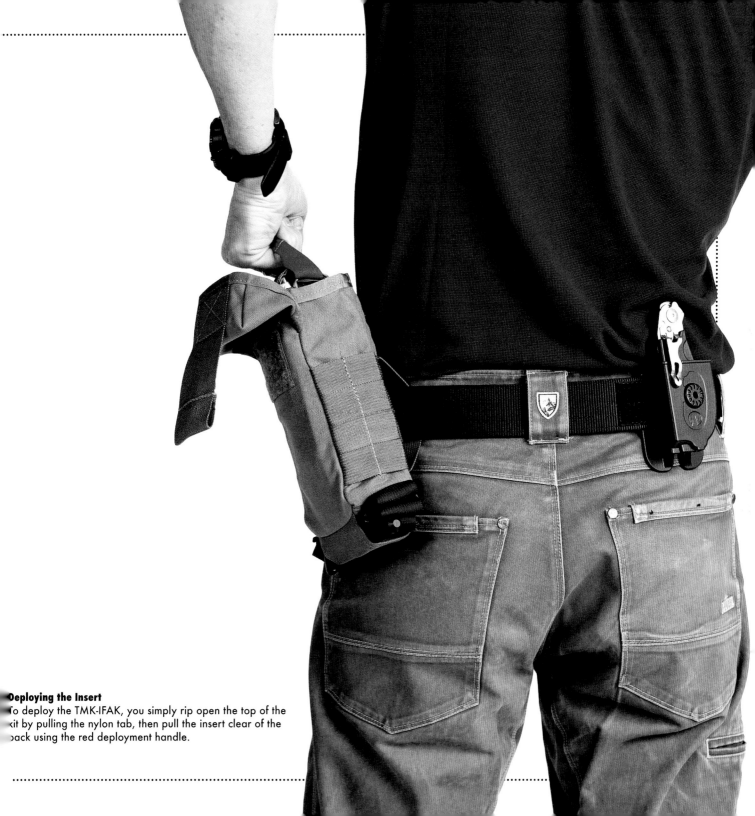

Deploying the Insert
To deploy the TMK-IFAK, you simply rip open the top of the kit by pulling the nylon tab, then pull the insert clear of the back using the red deployment handle.

Unlike the Gen 3 from Dark Angel, the TMK-IFAK contains a Bolin vented chest seal. While the vent reduces the chances of a tension pneumothorax, the Bolin package contains just a single chest seal. You would need two seals when dealing with entrance and exit wounds.

One other major difference with the Dark Angel kit is that the TMK-IFAK insert stores each of the items into its own elastic band or compartment. This allows you to access the tools individually, rather than by breaking the seal on a vacuum pack. You may also make your own substitutions. For example, you could swap the emergency bandage for the smaller version of the "H" bandage. You're also able to repack the kit yourself if you've used one or more items, such as the compressed gauze.

The innovation doesn't stop there — once you have configured the insert to your liking, fold it in half and secure it closed with the Velcro tab. The insert then slides into the outer pouch, with the red deployment handle sticking out the top. Close the top, attach it to your belt or backpack, and you're all set. If you need to deploy it, simply rip open the top of the kit by pulling the nylon tab, then pull the insert clear of the pouch using the red deployment handle. You'll notice that the insert is attached to the pouch with nylon webbing — this simple addition ensures that you never lose track of this lifesaving set of tools, even if you're under stress or under fire.

■ Universal Tourniquet Pouch

As shown on the previous page, the TMK-IFAK has a compartment under the pouch to store your tourniquet. But an IFAK is supposed to be about speed, and it takes a couple hands and a few seconds to release the tourniquet from the tight elastic band. If you'd like to access the tourniquet as fast as you can rip open a Velcro flap, you can add the Universal Tourniquet Pouch (UTQ) to the side of the TMK-IFAK as a dedicated compartment for any of the tourniquets profiled in Chapter 2. The UTQ can also be worn on the belt or any MOLLE compatible pack or pouch.

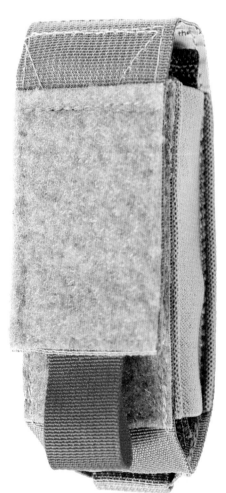

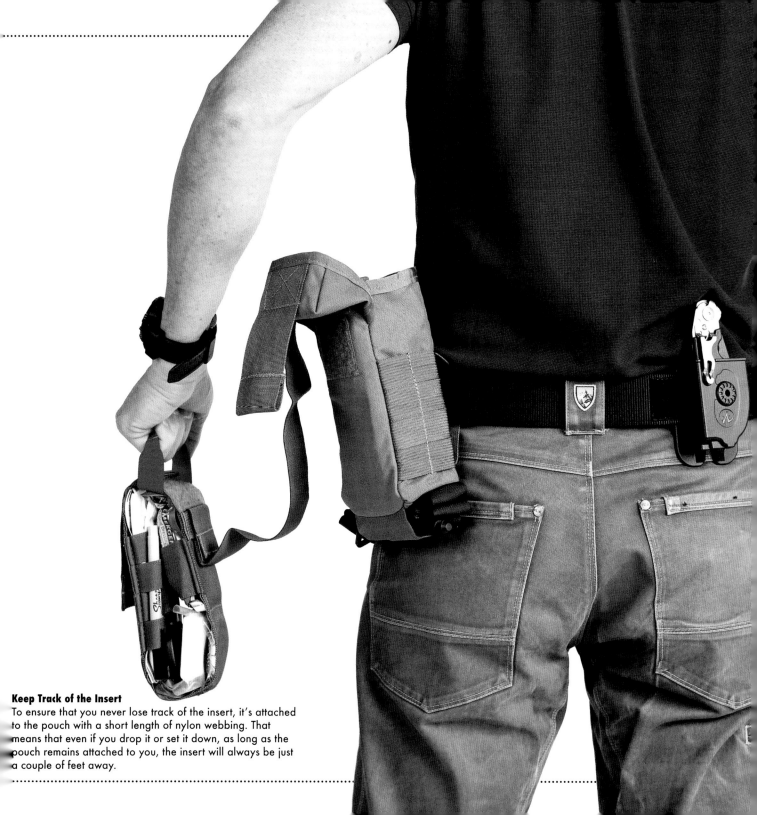

Keep Track of the Insert
To ensure that you never lose track of the insert, it's attached to the pouch with a short length of nylon webbing. That means that even if you drop it or set it down, as long as the pouch remains attached to you, the insert will always be just a couple of feet away.

CHINOOK TRAUMA MEDICAL KIT (TMK-IFAK)

Emergency Bandage
Like the Dark Angel Gen 3, the TMK-IFAK comes standard with an emergency bandage. But since each component has its own elastic band or compartment, feel free to swap out the emergency bandage for the smaller version of the "H" bandage if that's your preferred compression bandage.

Compressed Gauze
The TMK-IFAK comes with my favorite compressed gauze from H&H, which has multiple uses beyond packing a traumatic gunshot wound. You might be reluctant to tear open a vacuum-sealed insert to access your compressed gauze if it's just to wrap a twisted ankle — but since the TMK-IFAK stores every item separately, you won't feel so bad about it. Just don't forget to replace the gauze when you return from the field.

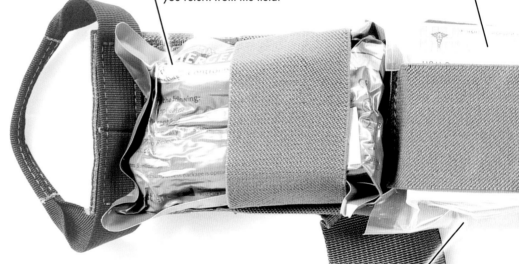

Fox Aluminum Eye Shield
While the Gen 3 packs a polycarbonate eye shield, the TMK-IFAK uses the aluminum eye shield from Fox. I replaced the standard eye shield with a version that has a soft cotton garter surrounding the outer perimeter of the shield. This makes wearing the shield a bit more comfortable for the patient.

Trauma Shears
Unlike the Dark Angel Gen 3, the TMK-IFAK stores its trauma shears within the insert, but since each item has its own separate compartment, accessing the shears is simple. In order to fit into the insert, these shears are slightly smaller than the standard size.

Nitrile Gloves
Like the Gen 3 from Dark Angel, the TMK-IFAK contains large nitrile gloves.

Bolin Chest Seals (1)
Like the HALO, the Bolin chest seal deserves top scores for its ability to adhere to blood- and sweat-slickened skin. In fact, after removing the plastic backing from the Bolin, you'll need to take great care that the seal doesn't become attached to you, your clothing, or anyone or anything around you before attaching it to the patient. The adhesive really is that good. Unlike the HALO, the Bolin has a vent which can help to reduce the chances of developing a tension pneumothorax. However, since the vent can become occluded with blood, you should still monitor your patient closely for signs of a tension pneumothorax (explained in Chapter 2) and "burp" the seal if those signs and symptoms develop.

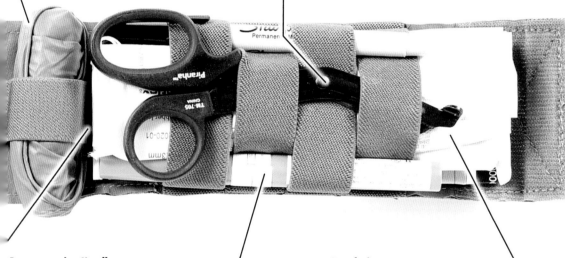

Decompression Needle
In its standard configuration, the TMK-IFAK comes with a decompression needle and nasal airway. If you're not trained in these devices, I suggest you pull them out of the insert and replace them with a SWAT-T tourniquet. If you're not familiar with the SWAT-T, check out page 203. It's an amazingly simple device with multiple uses.

Nasal Airway
See comment to the left.

Duct Tape
If you're wondering why duct tape would be in a trauma kit, it's because duct tape is the universal product used to fix broken items — or to field-improvise just about anything. In a pinch, thin strips of duct tape can fill in for adhesive sutures; it can be used to improvise a chest seal; it can repair a traction splint or contribute to a field expedient version, etc.

ADDITIONAL GEAR AND GADGETS

The gear I've outlined so far will meet the majority of your first-aid needs for both comfort and lifesaving situations. But if you happen to be a gearaphile like me, you may be interested in the additional items reviewed in this section — all of which are part of my personal emergency first-aid kits. I'll begin with a piece of personal equipment I mentioned in Chapter 1, namely, my favorite pair of trauma shears that go with me on every call.

Leatherman Raptor

It's fair to say that not all trauma shears are created equal and that's doubly true for the Leatherman Raptor. While standard trauma shears are made from pressed steel, the Raptors are cut from 420HC (high carbon) stainless steel. I've used other trauma shears to cut through jeans, boots and belts, but I recently used my Raptor to cut through a firefighter's multilayer bunker pants without breaking a sweat. I've even seen a demonstration of the Raptor cutting a quarter in half. Like all Leatherman products, the Raptor is a multitool. In addition to the shears, the Raptor includes a ring cutter, a seat belt cutter, a window punch and an oxygen tank wrench (always useful if you happen to be an EMT or paramedic and can't find the wrench on the ambulance). If you're unsure of when you'd need a ring cutter in an emergency situation, think back to our discussion of anaphylactic reactions in Chapter 3. Not only is that condition life threatening because it will cause swelling of the upper and lower airways and constriction of the bronchioles, it will also cause leakage of fluid from the capillaries and systematic blood vessel dilation. This leads to swelling of the extremities. If your patient's rings can't be removed before swelling occurs, they risk losing a finger or fingers unless the rings are cut off, *quickly*.

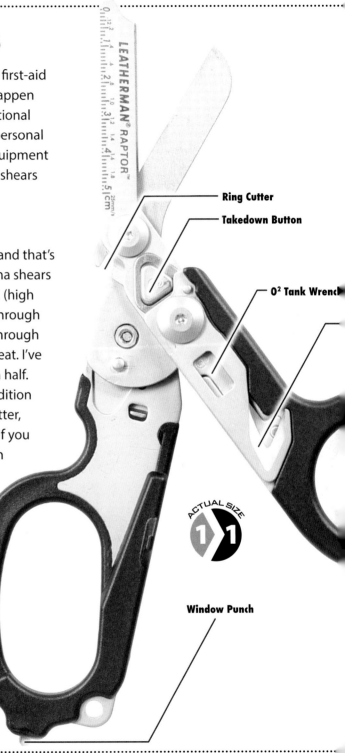

Ring Cutter

Takedown Button

O^2 Tank Wrench

ACTUAL SIZE 1 1

Window Punch

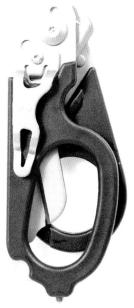

As if its powerful blades and multi-tool capabilities weren't enough, the Raptor also collapses into a small package by pressing the two buttons on opposite sides of the blades, then folding the blades inward. At that size, it easily slips into a pocket, a large IFAK or into the holster shown below.

Fold Out Seat Belt Cutter

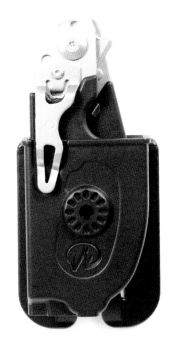

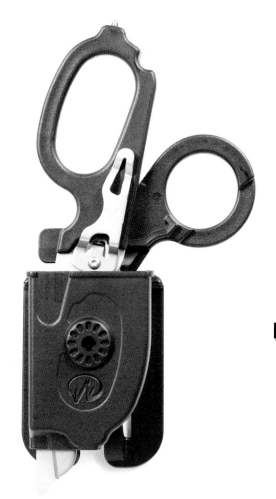

The holster (which is included) allows the blades to be inserted in either the open or collapsed position. In the collapsed position, the Raptor is held in place by the pocket clip, and in the open position, the Raptor is held in place by a retention lock on the backside of the holster. You must press this latch before you will be able to remove the Raptor (similar to a Level I holster for a handgun).

H&H Compressed Gauze

A standard addition to most trauma kits, it's worth including two or three extra packs of H&H compressed gauze in your small, medium or large first-aid kits. In its vacuum-packed package, the compressed gauze is just 3x2x1 — much smaller than a deck of cards. When unrolled, the compressed gauze is 4.5 inches wide by 12 feet long. In this image, the H&H compressed gauze is shown both in its vacuum pack and its unrolled state.

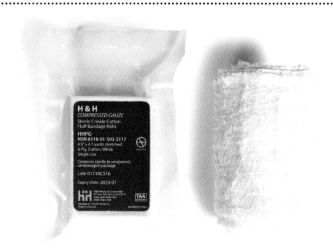

Benzoin Swabsticks

Benzoin dramatically increases the adhesiveness of sutures, tape and even moleskin, all of which seem to work their way loose, especially when you're in the field. Pre-apply to the areas where you'll be placing the adhesive dressing. The benzoin creates a tacky surface which keeps dressings from working their way loose. It may sound like a luxury item that isn't really necessary, but if your patient plans on remaining in the field after you've applied adhesive sutures, benzoin will ensure that the sutures remain in place and the laceration remains closed.

H&H Combat Eye Shield

The combat eye shield from H&H combines an aluminum Fox eye shield with a six-inch hydrogel disc, similar to an adhesive chest seal. Removing the backing of the shield and placing it over the injured eye replaces the need to wrap the injury in gauze and self-adhering tape over a traditional aluminum or polycarbonate eye shield. Like most of the products from H&H, the Combat Eye Shield is meant for those times when slow, methodical treatments aren't conducive to the harsh conditions that the victim and the rescuers find themselves in.

Rescue Essentials Tactical Ankle Medical Kit

I'm not a huge fan of ankle holsters when carrying a firearm, but I am a tremendous fan of this compact trauma kit from Rescue Essentials. The Tactical Ankle Medical Kit isn't going to store the same number of items as the IFAKs I profiled earlier, but the reality is, the larger the kit, the more likely it is that it gets left at home or at the station. For professionals (or nonprofessionals for that matter) who already carry too much on their belts, this ankle trauma kit might be the perfect answer. The pouch has three pockets and includes a SOFTT-W tourniquet, a 4-inch Israeli emergency bandage and a pair of nitrile gloves. With a small amount of space remaining, it's possible to fit in additional items such a pack of H&H compressed gauze or the SWAT-T tourniquet shown below.

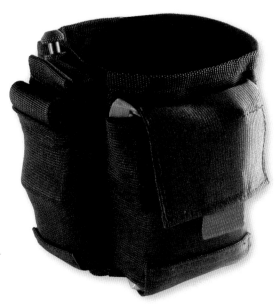

SWAT-T Tourniquet

After performing extensive research on the variety of tactical tourniquets and having seen them in action, I have to admit that I found it easy to dismiss this long piece of rubber as not being in the same league as modern wonders like the Ratcheting Medical Tourniquet. But as I started researching the SWAT-T and getting hands-on experience, I became a believer. Costing just 1/3 the price of the four tourniquets I profiled in Chapter 2, the SWAT-T has an amazingly simple method of deployment. It operates more like a compression bandage than a windlass or ratchet-driven tourniquet. Simply wrap the SWAT-T around the affected limb above the bleed and pull with enough tension on the elastic to make the rectangles in the pattern along the edge turn into squares. It's that simple. But, the SWAT-T is multitalented. You can also apply it with less pressure over a hemostatic dressing or surgical gauze to create a makeshift compression bandage. Alternatively, it can be applied loosely to hold an ice pack on a strain, sprain or fracture. Additional uses include acting as an occlusive wrap over a wet dressing covering an abdominal evisceration, as a swathe to stabilize a broken rib or any other use that you can come up with. Sometimes simple *does* make the most sense.

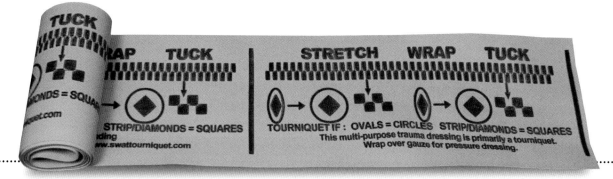

Pocket BVM (Bag Valve Mask)

For rescuers qualified to use a bag valve mask, the pocket BVM would make a valuable addition to a large- or medium-sized first-aid kit. It's no different in form or function to a standard BVM found on ambulances and in medic bags worldwide, but the innovative pocket BVM is packed into a cylinder about 25 percent the size of the fully deployed unit. When you open the top of the cylinder, the BVM pops up — kind of like a spring-loaded snake jumping out of a can of peanuts (and yes, I'll admit I jumped the first time I opened one). The BVM contains a full-sized mask, bag and even the oxygen connection that you'd expect to find. If you do purchase one and your curiosity gets the best of you, carefully unfold the collapsed BVM so that you'll know how to refold it to get it back into the cylinder.

A Space Saver

Like a gag snake popping out of a can, when the lid of the Pocket BVM is opened, a full-sized BVM pops out. Anyone who has ever carried a fully loaded medic bag knows how much space a BVM takes up. Too often, other important gear gets left out due to lack of space. The pocket BVM solves that problem by taking up just 25 percent of the space of a traditional BVM.

SAM Pelvic Sling II

In Chapter 2, I explained how to create a field expedient pelvic sling to stabilize an "open book" pelvic fracture. The innovators at SAM Medical (makers of the SAM Splint and SAM Chest Seal) have developed a commercially available pelvic sling that's easy to use and consistently provides the proper amount of pressure through the use of an "auto stop" buckle. Like the field expedient version, the SAM Pelvic Sling II slides under the patient's buttocks and aligns with the bony prominence on the sides of the hip — known as the greater trochanters (the knob-shaped end of the femur). The tension belt then slides through the auto-stop buckle until the buckle clicks (indicating that the proper pressure has been applied), and locks into place. Secure the belt with a Velcro attachment. In addition to being easy to use, SAM Medical designed the Pelvic Sling II to avoid overtightening or undertightening. A field expedient sling can either be applied with too much force, or too little force. That's not a concern with the Pelvic Sling II which will not allow a compression force greater than 33 pounds — considered to be an optimal amount of pressure for the average adult.

Of course, the average person doesn't need to carry this type of device in his or her emergency first-aid kit. But the SAM Pelvic Sling II would be a great addition to a gear lineup for first responders at any extreme outdoor recreational area including ski slopes, mountain climbing and extreme hiking areas and even white water rapids.

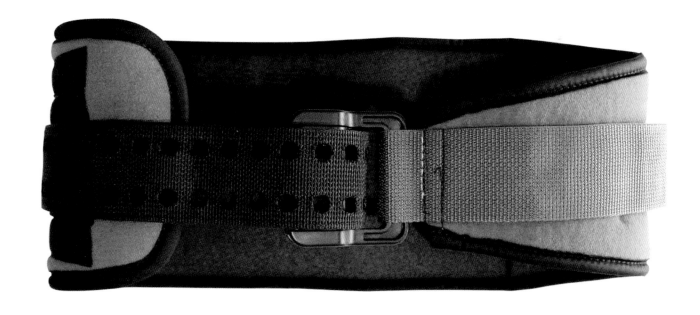

SO WHAT'S NEXT?

After finishing this book, you're probably wondering, "So what's next?" I'll leave you with a few suggestions.

Take a Class

While many of the skills in this book and our online course can be self-taught, several of the more technical skills require the experience of a skilled, experienced and patient instructor who can ensure that you're performing these lifesaving skills correctly. The American Red Cross and American Heart Association both sponsor classes ranging from hands-only CPR to conducting full-blown two-rescuer CPR. By taking a course from either

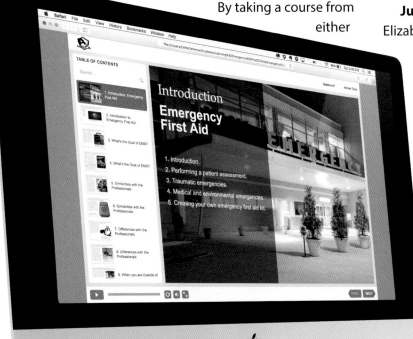

of these organizations (or through your local fire department, YMCA or school), you'll learn the proper way to recognize cardiac arrest and the proper way to deliver effective compressions and rescue breaths using a pocket mask or a NuMask. If you'd like to take a deeper dive into emergency first-aid training, I'd suggest taking a Wilderness First Aid course, sponsored by the National Outdoor Leadership School (NOLS).

Watch Some Videos

The American Heart Association has produced a number of excellent videos on the topic of cardiac arrest, heart attacks, stroke and more. My favorite videos include:

Just a Little Heart Attack — Comedian and actor Elizabeth Banks directed and starred in this video produced for the American Heart Association's "Go Red for Women" campaign. The video highlights the fact that many women ignore the signs of a heart attack until it's too late.

Hands-Only CPR With Ken Jeong — The American Heart Association is promoting "hands-only" CPR as a method of encouraging potential rescuers to jump into action when they might otherwise be squeamish at the thought of providing mouth-to-mouth resuscitation. The steps are simple. Step 1, call 911. Step 2, push hard and fast in the center of the chest at the same pace as the beat in the song, "Stayin' Alive." You shouldn't miss this educational (and hilarious) video.

Emergency First-Aid Fundamentals Online
The USCCA's online training offers important education to the millions of Americans ready to become their family's first responder. It's also great for those wanting to conduct pre-study before attending a live emergency first-aid course or who have already attended a course and are looking for a refresher.

Body Language — This video shows that body language can communicate a wide range of emotions; but one of the most important things it can tell you is if someone might be having a stroke. The American Heart Association and American Stroke Association are encouraging Americans to use the FAST acronym (as discussed in Chapter 3) to communicate the warning signs and symptoms of a stroke.

Learn Online

If you're not quite ready to take a live class but would still like to learn more about these important topics, you now have the option of taking the full USCCA Course, *Emergency First-Aid Fundamentals*, from the comfort of your own home. Within this online training, I'll act as your personal instructor. Three hours of video instruction in four lessons parallel the four chapters of this book. Unlike a traditional class, this online training allows you to take the course based upon your schedule and preferred pace. You can even rewind any portion of the course as many times as you'd like. The *Emergency First-Aid Fundamentals* course also contains dozens of video demonstrations which will allow you to explore these topics in more detail. At the end of each lesson, I'll test your knowledge with a highly interactive quiz. To learn more, visit USCCA.com.

Self-Led Training

As I mentioned earlier in this chapter, a large number of the skills explained in this book can be developed through self-led training, using the instructions in this book and a spare or two of any required tool or device. I suggest you start by learning to properly use a tourniquet, a compression bandage and explore the

many wonderful uses of a SAM splint. You can also practice applying the treatments for fractured ribs or a fractured pelvis on your friends or family. For a real challenge, construct the field expedient traction splint as explained in Chapter 2. While that splint is easy in theory, if you ever find yourself deep in the wilderness with a companion with a broken femur — and you've never moved beyond *reading* about that splint — your patient may be in for a long night. Practice not only makes perfect, practice makes *permanent*.

Conclusion

I hope that you've found the information in this book educational and that you can put it to good use if the need arises.

I'll end this book with a plea. One of my responsibilities with my local fire department is to lead our recruiting efforts, and I've seen first-hand the difficulty that suburban and rural departments have in filling their rolls — not to mention retaining trained individuals for more than a few years. If you've ever thought about becoming an EMT, a paramedic or a firefighter, stop thinking about it and visit your local department to ask if they're recruiting. Most departments offer full training for those skills. If you were to take this leap, I can guarantee you that it will be one of the most fulfilling things you'll ever do.

Finally, remember that *you* are your family's first responder. Take that responsibility seriously and stay safe.